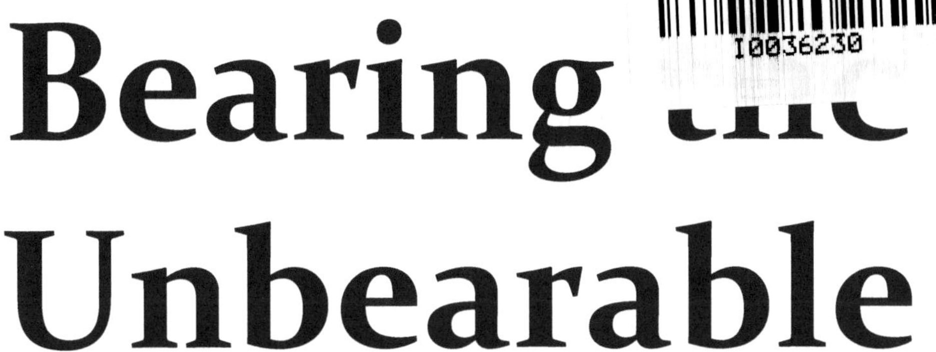

Bearing the Unbearable

Coping with Infertility and Other Profound Suffering

By Karl A. Schultz

NIMBLE BOOKS LLC

ISBN: 0-9788138-6-3

Last saved 2007-05-30.

Nimble Books LLC

1521 Martha Avenue

Ann Arbor, MI 48103-5333

http://www.nimblebooks.com

The cover and chapter artwork was contributed by Nick Parrendo, owner of Hunt Stained Glass Studios in Pittsburgh, Pennsylvania. For other artwork and background on Nick's stained glass work, visit his website: huntstainedglass.com.

Dedication

With love, to the one who accompanied me lovingly on the journey and shared in it in incomparable and unrepeatable fashion.

Karl

Acknowledgments

Thanks to my mother and father for their fertile love, prayers, understanding, and support in every way.

Love,

Karl

Other Works by Karl A. Schultz

The Art and Vocation of Caring for Persons in Pain. Mahwah, NJ: Paulist Press, 1994.

Becoming Community: Biblical Meditations and Applications in Modern Life New York: New City Press, 2007.

The Bible and You. with Loreen Hanley Duquin. Huntington, IN: Our Sunday Visitor, 2004.

Calming the Stormy Seas of Stress. Winona, MN: St. Mary's Press, 1998.

Christian Virtues and Values: Pope Paul VI. New York: Crossroad Publishing Company, 2007.

The How-To Book of the Bible. Huntington, IN: Our Sunday Visitor, 2004.

How to Pray with the Bible: The Ancient Prayer Form of Lectio Divina Made Simple. Huntington, IN: Our Sunday Visitor, 2007.

Job Therapy. Pittsburgh, PA: Genesis Personal Development Center, 1996.

Journaling with Moses and Job. Boston, MA: St. Paul Books & Media, 1996.

Nourished by the Word. with Fr. Andrew Campbell, OSB. Notre Dame, IN: Ave Maria Press, 1994.

Personal Energy Management: A Christian Personal and Professional Development Program. Chicago, IL: Loyola University Press, 1994.

Personal Energy Manager Rainbow Planner™. Pittsburgh, PA: Genesis Personal Development Center, 1996.

Where is God When You Need Him?: Sharing Stories of Suffering With Job and Jesus. Staten Island, NY: Alba House, 1992.

These books, plus audiotapes, CDs, and DVDs, are available from Genesis Center. The email address is karlaschultz@juno.com and the website is *karlaschultz.com*. The phone number is (412) 766-7545.

Contents

Table of Figures

Foreword

In my own family, and in my pastoral ministry, I have often encountered the deep suffering of those who desire to have children of their own and cannot. It is such an unexpected and unprepared for experience for married couples. Marriage preparations courses rightly spend much time on finances, fidelity, compatibility, dealing with in-laws and getting past the moonlight moments of being married. To my knowledge, however, little or no time is spent on what might be the most excruciating human experience—infertility. Whatever the accuracy of statistics, a surprisingly large number of couples have to face this reality with its accompanying pains: loss, expense of doctors, shame, embarrassing and intrusive questions from others, a sense of failure, anger, and envy to name just a few.

Karl Schultz convincingly depicts these and many more human sufferings caused by infertility. But his book differs profoundly in the ways it offers to transcend these sorrows—namely, by delving into the Bible and discovering how the inspired Word of God suffuses these sufferings with divine meaning.

It is this reflective, yet trenchant, inquiry into the riches of Sacred Scripture that separates Schultz's book from other works on the subject. Rather than look at infertility as a curse, the author places it among the many other human sufferings which afflict families and all humans. It is here that Schultz gives us a prayerful and knowledgeable reading of the history of God with humans. He shows the haunting language of love by which God woos and wins us. We reach the unbelievable love God found in the seeming failure of his Son, Jesus Christ. Innocent as he was, he learned obedience through what he suffered, and became the source of salvation for those who obey and follow him (cf. Hebrews 5: 8, 9).

I am sure that this book, and the strength it provides in its insights, in its invitations to put hard questions to oneself, in its wisdom to see suffering as a new call, will be of immense help to all those who suffer infertility, as well as to those who surround and love them. At the same time, Schultz challenges every sufferer to unite her or his suffering to Christ.

Reverend Timothy Fitzgerald, C.P., S.T.D.

Itinerant Preacher

The Inspirational Value of Artwork

Infertility, like all profound suffering, is a dimension of human experience in which actions can speak much louder than words, and a picture can be worth a thousand words. (However, some words must be said, hence the need for this book and communications between loved ones.) Accordingly, I have asked one of the greatest living religious artists, Nicholas Parrendo, President of Hunt Stained Glass Studios in Pittsburgh, to provide illustrations for the cover and each chapter.

Nick's pictures have an inspirational and catechetical as well as aesthetic appeal. Until the modern era, when literacy spread and books were more available, one of the main ways persons in the west received religious formation and education was through art. It remains an effective and pleasing mode of cultural and spiritual development in this world in which we are inundated with words and images designed to manipulate rather than uplift us.

The discussion of *lectio divina* in the Introduction also applies to art appreciation and assimilation. The reflections that accompany the pictures that precede each chapter are the fruit of my *lectio*, studies, and life experience.

Take in these pictures, observe how they communicate in images what the Bible describes in words and what you experience in life, and reflect upon the insights and emotions they evoke. Or, just enjoy them as a transition to each chapter or as works of religious art. Either way, art can be an edifying and elegant form of culture and communication:

"In approaching artistic masterpieces from whatever era, the mind is prompted to open itself to the mysterious fascination of the Transcendent, because a mysterious and unexpected spark of the Divine is present in every genuine artistic expression." (Pope John Paul II, address for the Jubilee Celebration for Artists, Friday, February 18, 2000).

Introduction

Bearing the Unbearable wrestles with two of life's most painful realities, the loss or diminishment of hope and the inability of human beings to fulfill their vocation, potential, and dreams. We will focus on perhaps the most poignant cause of this, infertility, but our discussion will include other major obstacles to fulfillment. There is an innate link between the futility of procreative and potential fulfillment efforts.

We will integrate western civilization's most famous infertility stories, those from the Bible, and particularly the Old Testament, with contemporary stories and your own.

Why I Wrote the Book

I wrote this book for two main reasons. First, I wanted to make the timeless insights and therapeutic applications of the Bible's infertility stories accessible to a wide audience. These can heal painful emotions and experiences, provide guidance on key decisions, and open up new ways of looking at your challenges and life as a whole. These stories transcend denominational boundaries and showcase universal emotions and experiences. They can truly be classified as world literature and every person's story.

Most books on infertility focus on emotional, social, financial, physiological, technological, homeopathic (natural remedies), and ethical issues. The spiritual aspect, which is closely linked to the others, has been largely overlooked, even though it is the aspect we have the greatest control over.

Second, I have dealt with infertility and other intimate suffering both personally and professionally, and have not found literary resources that addressed my experiences and concerns. I hope this book helps you to bear whatever is unbearable in your life, be it the lack or loss of children, setbacks, deprivations, or pain of any kind.

Who This Book is For

This book is particularly relevant for persons dealing with biological infertility, but it is also appropriate for anyone trying to bear up under other unbearable circumstances. It is meant for all persons struggling to give and affirm life in one way or another.

Bearing the Unbearable devotes attention to the most natural and literal manifestation of this challenge, infertility, in a way that encompasses other experiences of loss and deprivation. Both the Bible and our common language use infertility as a metaphor for the inability of persons and groups to achieve their goals.

The frustrations and challenges of infertility are similar to other intimate losses and deprivations, including various obstacles to living a full life. I refer to the latter as *functional infertility* because we're not able to function as we'd like.

For example, at fifty we are laid off and cannot use our talents in the workplace. A parent of three is abandoned by their spouse and has to raise and provide for their children largely by themselves. We graduate from college loaded down with student loans and are unable to get a job in our field. We'll discuss numerous common injustices in this book. By seeing the relatedness of different types of afflictions, we can be more understanding and compassionate towards ourselves and others.

Personal Experience

I approach the topic from the inside, quite aware of the subtleties and ambiguities involved. My struggles with life's deprivations have taught me that coping is more a matter of living the questions than of finding absolute answers.

No person's experience and perspective on such a subjective topic can be definitive. Because each person and situation is unique, I write in a dialogical, open-ended manner, offering familiar examples, customizable coping suggestions, and thought-provoking reflection questions.

Verbal and physical affirmation and poignant silence amid tragedy can speak eloquently. Through a balanced integration of stories, reflection, content, exercises, personal revelations, and humor, we can find meaning and direction amid the mystery of human impotence.

Getting Real and Getting Results

This book differs substantially from most self-help and inspirational books. It does not offer answers where there are none, nor does it paint a bleak picture rosy. It offers hope, inspiration, and practical guidance suited for the real world in which we live.

In this respect, it emulates the Bible, which approaches life in a realistic manner, unafraid to recognize its dark and gray aspects. Undeterred by sin and human weakness, the Bible emanates an underlying optimism and confidence in God and human beings, and a passion for life.

The Bible begins with the creation of life (Genesis) and ends with its consummation and perpetuation (Revelation). From beginning to end, it shows how to find joy, peace, and hope amid chaos. It is an ideal literary forum for confronting obstacles to fulfillment and discovering ways of transforming them.

We often hear the expressions "You can do whatever you set your mind to" or "You can get as far as you want in life." These have a grain of truth in them, but need to be qualified. Sometimes we can achieve our goals; other times obstacles force us to lower our sights and take alternate routes.

Authentic fulfillment of any dream or endeavor entails controlling what we can (free will, responsibility), and leaving the rest to God (providence), others (free will), and life (nature). This book offers suggestions for responding optimally to these factors in light of our afflictions.

Trying to give life rather than grief to self and others doesn't always produce desired results in the present, but it remains a healthy and harmonious way to live. Through the grace of God, your own efforts, and the support of others, may you bear up under your unbearable pressures, and bear fruit in the paths you travel.

Book Format

This book is composed and structured according to the ancient Christian model of holistic reading known as *lectio divina,* a Latin term meaning divine reading. It has its roots in the ancient Hebrew oral culture from which the Bible originated. It was developed and adapted by the early Christians, adopted by the desert fathers and mothers and their descendants, the monastic communities, most prominently the Benedictines.

As both professed religious and laypersons rediscover this accessible spiritual model, it is experiencing a modern rebirth. As can be deduced from its composition, it is an inclusive model appropriate for persons of all faiths.

Because it is an intimate dialogical practice that could be described as a spiritual version of sexual intercourse--a fitting analogy given both the Old and New Testament's use of marriage as a metaphor for God's relationship with his people-in a very real sense it transcends description. The only way to truly understand it is through experience.

However, for purposes of education, formation, and handing down among the generations, the following stages have been identified over the course of its transmission:

Reading and *listening*, in which the five senses are actively engaged. We read slowly, aloud or in a quiet murmur if feasible, and continue until we reach a word, phrase, verse, or image that strikes us, or perhaps brings a significant life experience to mind. The opposite of speed-reading, we engage a relatively small section of text, as the purpose is not to plow through it, but to savor it, as one does a grape or other piece of fruit, a metaphor used by the medieval monks who practiced this model faithfully.

Meditation is constituted by repetition of and reflection on the personally meaningful message derived from the passage, including relating the particular words, phrase, verse, or inspiration to other biblical passages or life experiences. The conscious and subconscious mind is prominent in this stage.

Prayer is the active component of dialogue with God. We share our response with God or others if practiced in a group setting. This is the affective dimension in the sense that we express our emotions and thereby discharge any toxic feelings, memories, or impulses; we convey how we are *affected* by the text or a life experience(s) which it brings to mind.

C*ontemplation* is the flip side of prayer and the receptive dimension of dialogue with God or others. Identified in Christian tradition as "simple presence", we wait silently on the Lord, opening ourselves to His message and the movement of the Spirit in our lives. In contemplation, the spiritual or unitive (the word religion comes from the Latin word *religio,* meaning to tie together or bind) faculty of human experience is most prominent, as we commune with God and perhaps others.

Historically, *action* was the last of the components to be explicitly articulated, though its role was implicit from the beginning. From the concrete, practical perspective of the Bible, it is the most indispensable component because it is where we practice our faith and bring it to life.

Further, since the traditional subject of *lectio divina,* God's word, cannot be identified exclusively with its normative expression (after Jesus, of course, cf. Jn 1:1-18; 1 Jn 1:1-4), the Bible, we should not make absolute distinctions between the practice of *lectio divina* on a written text or passage and *lectio divina* on a life experience. There is a natural fluidity and interaction between the two, as you will see in this book. I will frequently oscillate between life experiences and biblical texts as a way of grounding and balancing us in the truth of reality, found in both of the aforementioned.

We often discover biblical passages reborn in life experiences, as reflected in such vernacular expressions as the Good Samaritan and Prodigal Son. We read and reflect on the Bible and other spiritual texts in order to bring them to life.

A theological term coined in modern times, *praxis,* i.e., faith in action, captures the essence of this stage, which completes the holistic model by grounding it in life experience, reality, and human responsiveness.

The whole process is holistic (organic and natural, involving the whole person) and interactive rather than compartmentalized or methodical. The above descriptions are a map rather than a blueprint. Although the modular progression is descriptive of the typical way humans process significant stimuli and matters such as addressed in the Bible and this book, the process is ultimately spontaneous and natural rather than linear. Each time we practice *lectio divina* our experience (the process) may be slightly different, whether in direction, content / focus, speed, or intensity, which is natural and good because it is how we experience life, which is *lectio divina's* and the Bible's ultimate subject and context.

For further information on how the stages of *lectio divina* are played out in human interactions and communications and other activities (e.g., journaling, art appreciation and iconic devotion), see my books *The How-To Book of the Bible* and *How to Pray With the Bible,* both published by Our Sunday Visitor.

The ultimate testament to the efficacy of *lectio divina* is that we practice it naturally and experience its progressive, interactive stages even without cognizance of the terminology or model. Familiarity with its contents, flow, cohesiveness, and development over the centuries can only enrich and deepen our experience.

Perhaps the two words most descriptive of *lectio divina* are holistic and dialogue. It involves the whole person in an interactive, communication process, thereby helping us fulfill the first commandment (love of God with our whole self) and by relation, the second commandment, love of neighbor.

Although the activities comprising *lectio divina* permeate this book, they are communicated primarily implicitly, so as to facilitate a natural and fluid experience consonant with our circumstances and capacities.

Perhaps the most obvious manifestations of the *lectio divina* model are the reflection questions presented throughout the text. They are dialogical, open-ended prompts designed to stimulate personal application and assimilation, to make this book *your book.* You could spend the rest of your life contemplating the issues addressed in the questions and throughout the book, so don't feel obliged to answer them all. In the free-form, natural spirit of *lectio divina,* follow your reason, instincts, and the promptings of the Spirit in addressing them as circumstances merit.

Bible Translation

Biblical quotations and references are presented according to the New Revised Standard Version (NRSV) because of its clarity, literal accuracy, and ecumenical foundation and usage. Of course, you can use whichever Bible you prefer, and because the differences between most modern translations are not dramatic, the NRSV rendering of a passage will likely be similar to that of your translation.

Contacting the Author

I am interested in your comments and stories with regards to this book and topic. It will expand my horizons and deepen my understanding as I give presentations on infertility and related topics in a variety of health-care, support group, religious, and association environments. You can contact me in the following ways:

My email address is karlaschultz@juno.com, and my phone number is (412) 766-7545. The street address is Genesis Personal Development Center, 3431 Gass Avenue, Pittsburgh, Pa, 15212-2239.

Information on my speaking topics and other publications is available on my website, karlaschultz.com. This and my other books, audiotapes, CD's, and DVD's can be ordered using the above contact information.

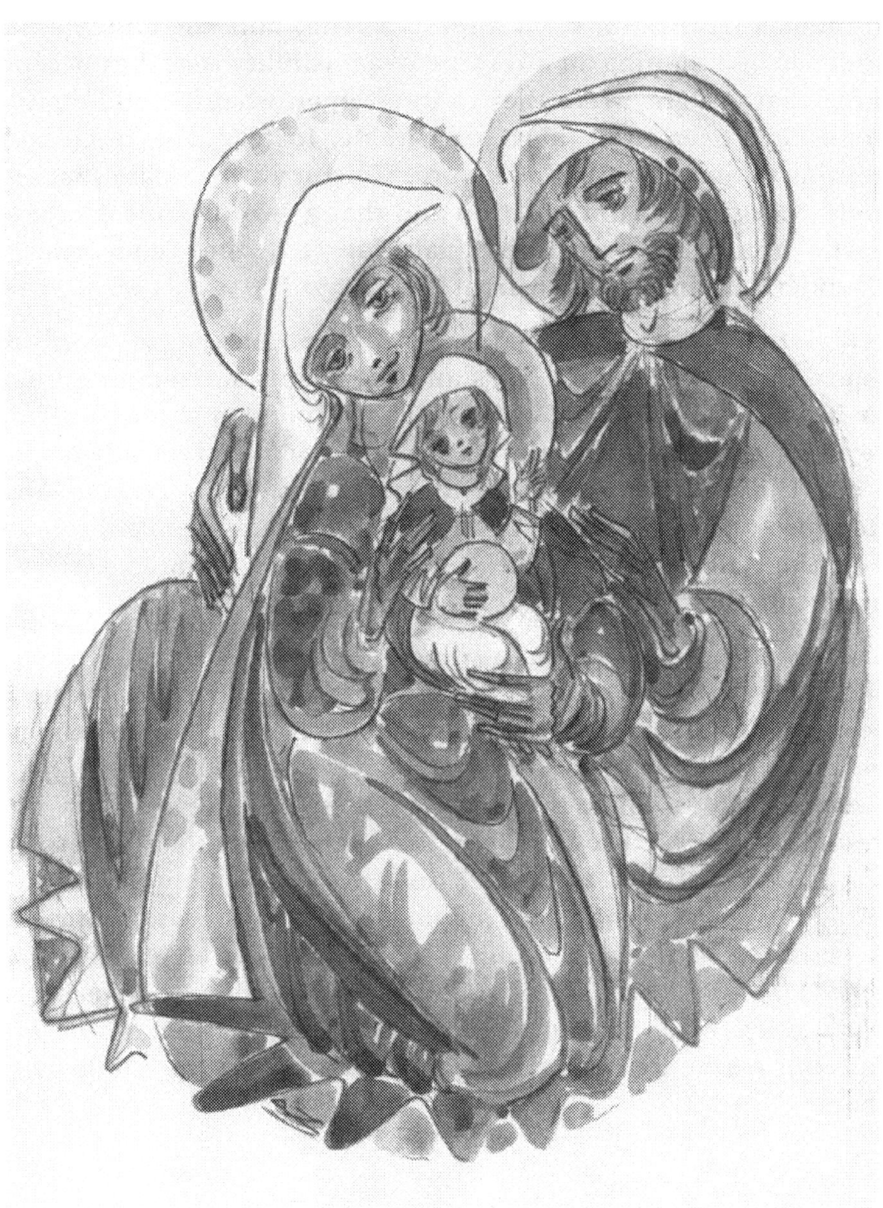

Figure 1. Mary, Joseph, and the baby Jesus.

An icon of Mary and Joseph constitutes a fitting beginning for this book's artwork for several reasons. They bore the unbearable in the sense of assuming an awesome responsibility that they accepted rather than sought. Were they to dwell upon what it could entail, it would have been even more unbearable. Instead, they focused on listening to and heeding God's word. Simeon warned Mary that Jesus would be a sign of contradiction and that a sword would pierce her heart. Yet, she remained faithful to the end, despite misunderstandings (cf. Lk 2:41-51; Jn 19:25-27).

Scripture records that Mary gave her consent in word and disposition (reflecting on Jesus and the events surrounding him in her heart; cf. Lk 2:19, 51), while Joseph responded through actions. We observe parallels with the way women and men typically respond to infertility. Women verbalize their feelings, often spontaneously, after deep reflection, while men take actions they deem appropriate, beginning, like Elkanah (cf. 1 Sam 1:8; see chapter six), with comforting their spouse.

Chapter one speaks of healing infertility through life-giving. While Mary gave life to Jesus, Joseph gave life to Mary by giving her the benefit of the doubt and extending mercy to her. In an insightful passage from his classic work, *Introduction to the Devout Life,* St. Francis de Sales comments that Joseph's example reminds us to presume good intentions on the part of our neighbor, unless they clearly demonstrate otherwise, and leave judgment to God. By opting for mercy rather than judgment, Joseph disposed himself to the message of the angel and assumed his role of guardian even before Jesus was born. Thus both Mary and Joseph bore Jesus in their hearts despite the lack of a physical consummation, which gives hope to us who are denied the joy of the fruit of the womb or our labors.

Chapter One

Healing Infertility Through Life-Giving

The best way to approach a problem is through the desired solution. For example, an approach to therapy referred to as solutions-focused counseling diverts our attention and energies from complaints and resentments and invites us to seek constructive resolutions. In the case of infertility and other losses and deprivations, the desired end is procreation and potential fulfillment. Fortunately, there is a resource, the Bible, that illuminates and integrates the two in an inspired manner.

A good care-giver is present to the one they serve, then gets out of the way. Permit me to step aside for the moment and spotlight the fundamental text in western civilization for understanding the source and purpose of life.

Beginning with Ideals and Moving to Reality

The first two chapters of Genesis are among the most uplifting and profound passages in world literature. Genesis presents two stories of creation, chapter one being written in the sixth century B.C., chapter two (beginning at verse 4) being composed in the tenth century B.C. They present universal and inspiring ideals from both God's (Gen 1) and humanity's (Gen 2) perspective, thereby providing a balanced and cross-generational synthesis.

Chapter three of Genesis, also from the tenth century, B.C. (sin and sorrow has a long history), the story with compelling symbols (e.g., the garden, the forbidden fruit, the snake) of human disobedience and its consequences brings us down to earth and serves as a realistic counterpoint to the ideals of Gen 1-2. Gen 1-2 teaches that it is natural for humans to seek to fulfill their procreative and developmental potential, and Gen 3 explains the roots of the difficulties we experience en route.

At this point in history, we need little reminder of the realities narrated in Gen 3. We need only pick up the newspaper or look around to reacquaint ourselves with life's brokenness. Reflecting on Gen 1-2 helps us rediscover our ideals amid the down sides of life, and approach even negative situations with a hopeful attitude.

The breadth of themes and insights in the first two chapters of Genesis necessitates that we stick to our focus. In this chapter, we will discuss the creation stories with respect to procreation and potential fulfillment. Chapter two will explore the link between the two.

Dual Dimensions of Infertility

By recognizing the interrelatedness of obstacles to vocation fulfillment, persons dealing with biological infertility will be better able to identify with persons struggling with functional infertility, and vice-versa. Couples experiencing both can recognize similar and cumulative effects, and take steps to avoid projecting their frustrations onto each other. Such awareness and solidarity help us bear each other's burdens, another ideal worth striving for (cf. Gal 6:2).

The first commandment of the Bible addresses both aspects of fertility: "Be fruitful and multiply, and fill the earth and subdue it; and have dominion over the fish of the sea and over the birds of the air and over every living thing that moves upon the earth" (Gen 1:28). We are told to procreate and exercise our potential. (Within the context of the Bible, dominion means creative and responsible stewardship, not exploitative domination.)

By exploring what this means in both the idyllic world of Gen 1-2 and in the real world of Gen 3 and today, we can develop a balanced approach to its application. Defining a problem, and breaking it into manageable aspects, is the first step in coping with it.

Dreams of an Ideal World

Wouldn't it be nice to get married knowing that if you wanted children you could have and afford them? Wouldn't it be nice if bearing and raising a child was not fraught with dangers and difficulties? Wouldn't it be nice to pursue a project or dream with reasonable assurance of fulfillment? Wouldn't it be nice to undertake challenging tasks and endeavors and not have to face disillusionment and frustration?

We live in a world where little is guaranteed. We cannot be assured of even the most basic things in life, such as waking up in the morning. Wise persons recognize this and live every day as if it may be their last, and treat others similarly.

Do I take life, myself, and others, particularly loved ones, for granted? How might I show my appreciation?

How might I renew my zest for life? How might I put little annoyances in perspective?

The Onset and Onslaught of Infertility

Clarence and Clarice had a smooth courtship and engagement, and a beautiful wedding and honeymoon. Then, the fireworks began. Clarence lost his job, and Clarice's company underwent a reorganization and her hours increased. They had names picked out for their five kids, but it soon became apparent that they might not be able to conceive one.

First came the visits to the gynecologist and urologist, then the fertility expert. How unpleasant and distressing things became, and so unexpected. Infertility can appear out of nowhere and have far-reaching effects.

Why would God give us a commandment that we would be unable to fulfill? Why would He implant a dream that might prove to be unattainable, and provide undesirable alternatives?

We can forget about getting absolute answers, at least in this life. However, we can wrestle with these questions and arrive at a more enlightened and peaceful attitude towards life, God, and ourselves. Our first step is to contemplate God's purpose in issuing the commandment, and the real world context in which we encounter it.

The Vocation of Procreation

One of the most beautiful and simple ways to understand procreation is to view it as God giving Himself children. He has arranged things so that He is dependent on us for this noble mission. He values our freedom and creativity so much that He makes even the most fundamental reality of human life, birth, hinge on our conscious choices. The nature of love, the highest virtue and the foundation of procreation and potential fulfillment, is that it is free.

What an awesome responsibility! Life-giving in any form, encompassing procreation, parenting, education, empowerment, facilitation, recreation, rehabilitation, and care-giving, is a vocation. Our response to life, from the womb to the tomb, makes a difference.

Contrary to depictions in popular culture, love is more than an emotion, impulse, or chemistry. It manifests itself in attitudes, decisions, and actions. Love seeks the good of others, and gives of itself towards that end. Love never keeps score (cf. 1 Cor 13:6).

1 Cor 13 is a practical and profound description of the dynamics of love. Through the use of verbal expressions (see the passage presented below), it conveys not only what love is, but what love does. Reflecting on this passage and considering if you meet its ideals is a step towards rekindling love. Replace the word "love" with your name and observe how it sounds and feels:

> "Love is patient; love is kind; love is not envious or boastful or arrogant or rude. It does not insist on its own way; it is not irritable or resentful; it does not rejoice in wrongdoing, but rejoices in the truth. It bears all things, believes all things, hopes all things, endures all things" (1 Cor 13:4-7).

Am I approaching my procreation and potential fulfillment efforts in a spirit of love?

If frustrations, distractions, hyperactivity, and self-absorption have eroded my love, am I willing to recapture it? What steps will I take?

Primitive Insights

As evidence of the crucial role humans assume in procreation, the Bible describes the birth of the first human being, Cain, through the lens of the mother, Eve: "I have produced a man with the help of the LORD" (Gen 4:1).

Interestingly, the role of the man goes unmentioned, while God's pivotal involvement is acknowledged. Likewise in life we find most mothers conscious of God's role in their maternity, while the man's role naturally gets pushed into the background

Heavenly and Human Help

Let's focus on Eve's description of God's involvement as being one of "help." This term was used in Gen 2:18, 20 to describe the mutuality of husband and wife, and in a broader sense, the genders. Marriage is meant to be constituted by mutual help and support, i.e., teamwork. God is an integral part of the marriage equation, for in the most fundamental act of life-giving, He is acknowledged by the mother as a helper even more essential than her husband. After all, God is the source and sustainer of life.

God's role of helper extends far beyond procreation. We recognize this in common parlance, inviting others to pray for us and invoking God's help in our pursuits. Even persons skeptical of God's existence or efficacy petition God's help during crises.

If I view God as a helper rather than as an adversary or bystander during my procreation and potential fulfillment efforts, I am more likely to display a hopeful and cooperative attitude. I will waste less energy fighting God and life, and avoid the stifling guilt and resentment that accompanies it.

In my procreation or potential fulfillment efforts, do I view God as a helper, adversary, or onlooker? How does this affect my attitude and actions?

How might I change my perspective so that I cooperate more fully with God and fight life less?

The Mystery of Providence

When we invite God's help, we cannot program it. In the Bible, the qualifier to petitions for divine help is "as God wills." We want absolute control, but we have to settle for substantial influence.

We often hear the expression "God answers all prayers, but sometimes says no." A more accurate observation is that God responds to prayers in His own time and way:

> "For my thoughts are not your thoughts, nor are your ways my ways, says the LORD. For as the heavens are higher than the earth, so are my ways higher than your ways and my thoughts than your thoughts" (Isa 55:8-9).

There is no comprehending the mystery of providence (God's caring involvement in the world). At best, we can have intuitions and insights, such as when we perceive God's hand in our affairs. For example, events unfold that we are convinced reflect divine providence. We perceive that He is trying to teach, develop, and heal us, as well as help us in practical situations.

Discovering God's Initiative

The fundamental religious experience is discovering God's initiative in our life. It's particularly crucial for surviving difficult times, when we feel as if He has abandoned or rejected us, or worse, is punishing us.

Everyone experiences God's presence in their life in a different way. For most people, it is subtle. Few folks have direct encounters like Moses at the burning bush (cf. Exod 3).

I experienced God's initiative in my life in a particularly compelling way when I first began writing and speaking in 1988. Starting out was difficult, and amidst my turmoil I came across a little known modern spiritual classic entitled *Through Moses to Jesus* by Carlo Martini, S.J. (Ave Maria Press). This book showed how Moses' experience at the burning bush translates in a unique way to each of us. I subsequently incorporated Martini's insights in a book entitled *Journaling with Moses and Job* that integrates excerpts from the aforementioned with practical pointers on journaling, personal development, and inner healing.

Drawing on Jewish and Christian tradition, the author, a world-famous biblical scholar and church leader, discussed why the pivotal stage in spiritual development is the discovery of God's initiative in our life. It shifts our focus from what we do for God to what He is doing for and with us. This inspires us to respond by sharing His love with others:

> "We love because he first loved us. Those who say, "I love God," and hate their brothers or sisters, are liars; for those who do not love a brother or sister whom they have seen, cannot love God whom they have not seen" (1 Jn 4:19-20).

Up to that point I had been devoted to my faith, but with an emphasis on what I had to do to earn and maintain God's love. What a revelation it was to rediscover that God's love was mine prior to and independent of any efforts on my part, and that He was actively involved in my life. Suddenly events took on a transcendent meaning, and I began to notice subtle indications of God's hand in my life.

Did I hear God whispering in my ear? No. Did I have a deep emotional or physical experience of His presence? No. However, looking at events in my life through the eyes of faith, I began to discover positive patterns and developments that I might be able to explain on a natural level, but for which the more fitting explanation was spiritual.

For example, a small opportunity that I was only partially responsible for procuring would open up. Or I'd have an encounter that gave me a message that I needed to hear. A common term for such experiences is providential. When people say "this was meant to be" or "there is a reason why this happened", they are usually referring to providence. Most people see God behind these events, while others ascribe it to fate, destiny, the universe, or human energies.

Conversely, even negative developments would reveal a silver lining. For example, I would encounter a disagreement or major inconvenience and some positive lesson would emerge. Of course, there are many times where God doesn't seem present, or I don't understand the meaning of a negative event, but that doesn't mean that God isn't involved. Part of the challenge of faith is to believe that God is working even when it is not apparent.

God's Initiative Amid Afflictions

The discovery of God's initiative is particularly relevant when we are dealing with infertility and other obstacles to fulfillment. The overall message we are getting from life may be negative, but we should not confuse that with God's mindset. The Bible is filled with agonizing over the prosperity of the wicked and the difficulties of the just (cf. Ps 31; 37; 44; 69; 73; Jer 20; Job 24; Hab 1; Wis 2).

When we are trying to cope constructively with our situation, we can receive consolation and guidance from paying attention to God's initiatives in our life. Most of us are familiar with the expression "when God closes one door, He opens another." We want to be particularly receptive to "divine signs" (manifestations of His initiative in our life and pointers regarding the direction He wishes us to take). We can discern God's presence and activity through prayer, spiritual reading, journaling, dialogue with God and other spiritual persons, reflection on life experiences, and an open heart.

Jill and John found out that they were going to have difficulty having a child. Crushed, they went through a period of decreased communications and alarming distancing. Finally, they went to see a therapist.

Jill and John discovered that each had unresolved childhood issues that were becoming impediments to their union. Had they conceived a child, this would likely have gone unnoticed, only to manifest itself during the stressful period of child-raising. Jill and John were relieved that things had transpired such that they could build a more stable foundation for their marriage prior to beginning a family.

What experiences have you had of a seemingly negative event turning out to have positive consequences?

Communicating with God Regarding His Initiative

Each night I write in my journal the ways I experienced God in my life that day. It could be very mundane things or it could be an uncommon occurrence. Either way, my journaling observations affirm both His presence in my life and my constructive response to life's opportunities. My entries often resemble each other, as God usually works in my life in a consistent, subtle way. Most of us would be overwhelmed by frequent "burning bush" experiences. Moses' encounters with God were so intense that his face lit up, thereby requiring a veil so as not to scare the Israelites (cf. Exod 34:29-35).

I don't have proof of God's direct involvement, nor do I give such a great deal of thought. God is usually not that transparent. However, believing that God is the underlying source of all the good that happens in my life, I can freely ascribe to Him such occurrences and thank Him (cf. Jas 1:12-18). This takes the focus off of me and inspires me to view God as working with rather than against me.

Knowing that God accepts me helps me make constructive changes without thinking I'm bad or being rejected. Conversely, the misguided notion that God opposes me fuels resentment and negativity. In the Old Testament, God is frequently described as our rock and helper. In the New Testament, the Holy Spirit is described by Jesus as our advocate (cf. Jn 14:16, 26; 15:26; 16:7), and Jesus also is referred to as our advocate (cf. 1 Jn 2:1). Accordingly, we can view God as our advocate and try to be an advocate for ourselves and others. This inspires a positive approach to developments in life. Conversely, the Hebrew word for the evil spirit, *satan,* means accuser or adversary, and the word "devil" means slanderer. Thus when we tear down ourselves or others, we are not focusing on God's initiative, but on our private agenda, and may be acting as unwitting accomplices of the devil.

When I am impeded from fulfilling my potential or denied opportunities that are rightfully mine, I express my frustrations to God and listen to His response. He typically manifests Himself and His will through such stimuli as an inspirational or instructive Bible passage, a peaceful revelation during prayer, or through some event or interpersonal encounter. In any event, I continue doing my part to fulfill my potential, confident that God is pleased with my efforts and will use them to accomplish His will.

Do I believe that God takes the initiative in my life?

In what events have I felt God's presence?

How might I make God's initiative a more central part of my outlook, faith, and activities?

The Mystery of Procreation

If we can only partially comprehend God's activities in daily life, we can hardly expect to understand His will in one of the most fragile and mysterious of quests, that of procreation. Just as God's help is no panacea or guarantee in our efforts to fulfill our potential (the second half of the commandment in Gen 1:28), so His presence and support does not make us immune to the difficulties of conception, pregnancy, and child-rearing. Gen 3:16 blames the difficulties associated with the vocation of wife and mother on the disruption introduced into creation by human sinfulness:

> "To the woman he said, "I will greatly increase your pangs in childbearing; in pain you shall bring forth children, yet your desire shall be for your husband, and he shall rule over you."

Of course, not all infirmities and obstacles can be directly traced to sin. The author of Genesis was familiar in only a rudimentary way with natural causes and other mitigating factors in life. He lived in a God-centered, primitive world where things were explained on a moral and theological rather than scientific basis. The point of the text is that God did not intend for life to be as painful as it is. Human beings introduced disorder through disobedience, thus causing a series of chain reactions, such as the struggles between humanity and nature signified by the growth of thorns and thistles (cf. Gen 3:17-19).

We influence the conception, child-bearing, and child-rearing process, so we should not look to God alone for help. We have to help ourselves and each other. The secret of inner peace and prudential actions lies in finding a happy medium between dependence on providence and responsible actions. This is captured in the spiritual maxim: "Pray as if everything depends on God, act as if everything depends on you."

Do I need to grow more in trust or responsibility? What steps might I take to achieve a better balance?

The Challenge of Obedience

The fragilities and ambiguities in the procreation and potential fulfillment process derive from the laws of nature and human freedom, and the mystery of providence. Through science and spirituality we can gain insights into procreation, but our knowledge is only partial (cf. 1 Cor 13:8-12). Where does this leave us with respect to God's commandment to bear children and to exercise our potential in a constructive manner? How do we proceed prudently and peacefully given our imperfect understanding and the many obstacles in our path?

Here we come a biblical value repulsive to most modern Westerners. A pre-eminent value in most civilized cultures until modern times, obedience has been superseded by a one-sided understanding of freedom as license.

Ancient societies presumed obedience. There were significant consequences for disobedience. It was considered virtuous rather than a sign of weakness. In our times, disobedience often leads to fame and fortune, frequently followed by a book deal. Yet, obedience remains essential to redeeming our experience of infertility or other afflictions.

The word obedience comes from the Latin *ab audire*, to listen to. In our noisy, fast-paced world, we have compromised our ability and willingness to listen to each other. One of the fundamental characteristics of love is the willingness to listen to our loved one, to be present to them as they express themselves.

Accepting our Best

The Bible's first commandment, to procreate and develop creation and ourselves (cf. Gen 1:28), was given in the ideal context of a world without sin. The Bible is decidedly non-speculative. It provides no clues as to whether procreation would have been automatic or unimpeded in a world unmarred by sin. Neither does it reveal whether realizing our potential in a perfect world would have been free of obstacles and frustrations. Since none of us have experience of a perfect world, we cannot know this.

Because we live in a broken world, we must insert the word "try" into the Bible's first commandment. We can't control whether we conceive and bear a child, nor can we effectively micro-manage our potential fulfillment. Some factors are out of our hands. All we can do is our best.

We have to work towards satisfying ourselves with best efforts. Both nature and nurture (environmental influences) incline us towards results, the satisfaction of our objectives. Who undertakes a significant activity with ambivalence towards the outcome?

We may not like certain results, but virtue and maturity enable us to make the best of them (responsible receptivity) rather than slip into passivity, self-pity, or fatalism.

Do I accept my and my loved ones' best efforts, or do I insist on perfection? What happens when I choose the former? The latter?

What are my internal and external obstacles to satisfying myself with best efforts? How might I overcome these?

Do I trust God? Why or why not?

Pursuing Positive Alternatives

When our conception and potential fulfillment efforts fail to bear fruit, we have to courageously pursue alternate ways of giving life, without giving up on our primary goals. Another application of Gen 1:26-28 is that God has given us the creativity and resourcefulness to adapt to circumstances.

How often we hear of couples who adopt after a long period of infertility, then end up having one or more natural children! Does this ensue from the relaxed nature of their efforts courtesy of the pressure being off and their choosing a constructive response—who knows?

God has not provided a blueprint for procreation and potential fulfillment. The Bible articulates values and directives for living justly and fulfilling God's will, but we have to discern how to apply them. Each person and circumstance merits its own response. The Holy Spirit can help us discern how we should apply God's guidelines, but He does not eliminate ambiguities or risks. This is part of being human. He promises to be with us as we face these gray areas and the accompanying negative consequences.

If necessary, what positive alternatives to my/our preferred path towards fulfillment might I/we pursue?

Listening to God

We can approximate what it means to listen to God, in particular the Bible's first commandment, by considering what it means to listen to each other. Listening implies a sincere willingness to please our partner, to bring them peace, joy, and fulfillment. We want what is good for them, and try to bring it about. With God things differ slightly, because we obey Him more for our sakes than for His, since God always wills what is good for us.

Responsive listening to God requires us to show good faith and concern, to take steps to bring about what He desires. Our words and actions work together towards this end. This implies an openness to and celebration of life, a desire and commitment to bring it about and affirm it from the womb to the tomb.

From a moral and developmental standpoint, taking care of the elderly is one of the most dignified and socially necessary potential fulfillment activities. Paradoxically, we give without expectation of reward, yet learn and receive much from the elderly.

In previous generations, taking care of the elderly was a social obligation. The commandment to honor your mother and father includes taking care of them in their old age:

> "Those who honor their father atone for sins, and those who respect their mother are like those who lay up treasure.
>
> ...My child, help your father in his old age, and do not grieve him as long as he lives;
>
> even if his mind fails, be patient with him; because you have all your faculties do not despise him. For kindness to a father will not be forgotten, and will be credited to you against your sins; in the day of your distress it will be remembered in your favor; like frost in fair weather, your sins will melt away" (Sir 3:3, 12-15).

We should affirm ourselves for trying to give life in whatever way is open to us. Leaving the results to God is a mature manifestation of trust and obedience, an act which pleases Him. As Mother Teresa of Calcutta frequently observed, God doesn't ask us to be successful, but faithful.

Holy men and women in the Bible and down through the centuries have experienced countless setbacks, doubts, and disappointments, but they persevered in their obedience and bore fruit according to God's will. We may not understand how we are bearing fruit, but we can trust that if we try, God will bless our efforts in His own way and time:

"The point is this: the one who sows sparingly will also reap sparingly, and the one who sows bountifully will also reap bountifully. Each of you must give as you have made up your mind, not reluctantly or under compulsion, for God loves a cheerful giver. And God is able to provide you with every blessing in abundance, so that by always having enough of everything, you may share abundantly in every good work. As it is written, "He scatters abroad, he gives to the poor; his righteousness endures forever." He who supplies seed to the sower and bread for food will supply and multiply your seed for sowing and increase the harvest of your righteousness" (2 Cor 9:6-10).

Do I want to listen to God amid my current difficulties, knowing that His message may require me to change and let go of negative energies, attitudes, and behaviors? It is easy to become comfortable holding on to resentments and self-pity.

What listening activities am I disposed to: e.g., prayer, meditation, journaling, communing with nature, spiritual reading, dialogue with a spiritual guide or fellow believer(s)?

Do I believe that God will eventually come through? Am I willing to present my doubts or frustrations to God and wrestle with Him and them?

Mixed Signals on Children

Let us now reflect on the intended fruits of our efforts. Modern society has a paradoxical attitude towards children. On one hand, we allocate billions to their development, and undertake stringent measures to protect them. At the same time, we undermine our efforts by whittling away at parental jurisdiction and authority and exposing children to the basest forms of entertainment and education. We thereby make them more vulnerable to their most dangerous enemies: themselves (naiveté, inexperience, foolhardiness, unbridled peer pressure) and exploitative adults.

From our modern materialistic perspective, children are first a commodity and an expense. Children were viewed differently in pre-modern times because they were not only mouths to feed, but hands to help. Children were an economic asset, and family life was much less children-centered than today.

Infertility's Societal Dimension

From a social justice standpoint, infertility is complicated by the fact that some persons do not have the resources to get the best treatments and to explore all options (e.g., adoption). Woe to society for condoning wanton luxury for a minority while depriving many of a reasonable possibility of a dignified family life. Woe to society for sanctioning and even glorifying exorbitant entertainer, athlete, and executive salaries. Woe to political and economic leaders for tolerating communally detrimental takeovers and consolidations. These and other manifestations of greed have left many couples wondering whether they will be able to provide economically for their children.

Infertility is not an issue in isolation. It is a community problem, and requires community participation in the solution. That children have become an economic and social burden is a sad reflection on society.

What can I do to address infertility on a social justice level? Examples include avoiding greed, exercising social sensitivity in business decisions, and working for the interests of children and would-be parents.

Reverence for Life

Children are a gift from God and a special way that humans participate in the life-giving process. Couples struggling with infertility recognize the giftedness of children in a special way. Deprivation is a painful but poignant teacher.

One of the lessons of infertility is that God's gifts are at His disposal. We can prove ourselves unworthy of them by taking them for granted or by being ill-disposed to receive and nurture them.

We live in a presumptuous, entitlement-oriented, society which views humanity and its progress as the measure of all things. This differs considerably from the biblical and spiritual perspective, where everything is gift, beginning with life.

In the Bible, only God has dominion over human life. This underlies the severe prohibitions against murder (cf. Gen 9:5-6) which precede God's post-flood restatement of the procreation commandment (cf. Gen 9:7). We have defiantly appropriated this prerogative for ourselves not only through willful acts of violence but through dehumanizing culturally-sanctioned practices such as euthanasia, capital punishment (innocent people have been put on death row before being exonerated while some have even been executed), and abortion. These are the opposite of life-giving and a brutal disposing of the vulnerable.

Viewing the issue from a positive standpoint, we can affirm that all outreach to the elderly, impressionable teen-agers, expectant mothers, and even criminals (God is their ultimate judge, and some are wrongly convicted), to name just a few vulnerable constituencies, is a participation in the creative process of life-giving entrusted to us by God at the beginning of creation.

Each Act and Person Matters

I have had the opportunity to work with teen-age boys at a residential treatment facility. Many have run afoul of the law. Some have been convicted unjustly. Many have no advocates. Sometimes the staff and administration of their treatment facility do not stand by them. Virtually all come from troubled families.

There are few more rewarding experiences in life than spending time with these children. They are far more appreciative of outreach than many adolescents I know from stable families in the suburbs. You can't buy the warm feeling that comes from knowing that you let just one person know that you care. Their smiles, handshakes, hugs, and teasing speak volumes.

My experience there reminds me of my favorite Bible verse—Jesus' response to the just at the last judgment: "Amen, I say to you, whatever you did for one of these least brothers of mine, you did for me" (Mt 25:40, New American Bible).

Jesus isn't into big numbers. This verse epitomizes the particularity of true spirituality: "whatever you did"— each act counts, and "for one of"—

each person counts. Politicians and visionaries have grand plans, which have their place, but there is no substitute for one-on-one outreach. This is the foundation of potential fulfillment, because you further both your own and your neighbor's potential. What is more particular and individual than the birth of a child or multiple births?

How might I live a more particularist life that values individual gestures and persons?

Am I willing to be particularly kind to myself, doing little things as a reminder of my dignity? I cannot give what I don't have.

Do I believe that when I do good to others or myself, particularly when vulnerabilities are involved, that I do good to God? Mother Teresa lived by this code, and she surely actualized her potential.

The only enduring answer to the mystery of suffering is to do good to those who suffer, including ourselves. From this perspective, it is unacceptable for men and women who are unable to exercise their procreative or developmental potential to hang their heads or view their affliction as punishment. The opposite is true: affirming their worth in the face of punishment helps them identify with Jesus, and reveal him to others.

Breaking the automatic association of suffering with punishment was another point emphasized by Mother Teresa. One of her most popular stories was of an encounter with a dying woman, to whom she said "Jesus is kissing you from the cross." The woman responded: "Mother Teresa, tell Jesus to stop kissing me."

When we are in the midst of suffering, it pleases God when we ask Him to lift His heavy hand from us. What loving parent is not drawn to mercy when administering appropriate corrections?

Do I believe and accept that God occasionally has a heavy hand, or do I attribute such circumstances to life and human freedom?

What experiences have I had of God's or life's heavy hand?

When I brought my anguish to God, what was my experience of His or my own response?

Am I willing to perseveringly petition God for mercy, like the widow before the corrupt judge (cf. Lk 18:1-8)?

The Cost and Rewards of Service

It has been my consistent experience that people who endeavor to serve God and their fellow human beings are often treated harshly. Abraham (see chapter three) and Moses are profound biblical examples. After all Moses did for God and the Jewish people, he was denied entry into the promised land, and his burial place remains unknown (cf. Deut 34:4-6).

Interestingly, in the very next verse the Bible affirms the link between suffering, service, and potential fulfillment: "Moses was one hundred twenty years old when he died; his sight was unimpaired and his vigor had not abated" (Deut 34:7).

The man who was rewarded with the rare title "servant of the Lord", the molder and glue of the Jewish people and the Torah (the first five books of the Bible), who suffered excruciating trials and who weakened on occasion (cf. Num 20:7-12; Deut 1:22-38), the one whose exhortation to choose life is a mantra for this chapter and book (cf. Deut 31:15-20), died at 120 in the pink of health (with vision and vigor intact). Moses offers dramatic testimony that a life-giving vocation fosters wellness and potential fulfillment for the self and others.

In his leadership vocation Moses had to redirect his procreative energies. The Bible mentions two sons he had before returning to Egypt (cf. Acts 7:29). The Bible relates a touching reunion of Moses and his family in Exod 18:1-12. Like Abraham, Moses experienced impairments of family life because of his divine commission, which he resisted initially (cf. Exod 3:7-4:17). As we will see in chapter three, Abraham likewise had his doubts.

Since life is God's initiative, He chooses us and sets the rules, but we can always say no. Pope Paul VI (1897-1978) often prefaced his comments about God's demands with "whether we like it or not." This captures the reality of the occasional unpleasantness of our life-giving vocation.

When we suffer fertility and potential fulfillment obstacles, we are in good company, though in the heat of hurt that realization hardly compensates. Only through reflection, prayer, and patient trust in providence can we take consolation from our solidarity with others.

Female Firebrands

As we will see, infertile women have a unique relationship with God in the Bible. They also know how to stand up to their man. Of course, such qualities are not limited to biblical times. Two prominent celibate women from the Middle Ages exemplify this in an inspiring manner.

In 1970, St. Catherine of Siena was the second woman to be proclaimed a doctor (sublime and authoritative teacher of Catholic doctrine) of the Catholic Church. She made her mark in the 14th Century in part by successfully urging Pope Gregory XI to move the papacy back to Rome from Avignon, France. Though her education was limited and she died at a young age, Catherine was extraordinarily influential in affairs of church, state, and society.

The first woman named doctor of the Church and one of the greatest teachers of prayer in Christian history, St. Teresa of Avila, was likewise no shrinking violet. In her exercise of righteous wisdom, she went higher than Catherine. She told off the pope's boss.

En route to one of the convents she oversaw, she was unceremoniously thrown from her carriage and covered with mud. Apparently having learned from the matriarchs and holy women of the Bible (including Job's newly childless wife, who advised Job to curse God in response to his unconscionable afflictions; cf. Job 2:9), she was not hesitant to let God know how she felt: "God, if this is how you treat your friends, it is no wonder you have so few of them." I believe He'd agree.

Prayer and Passion

Just as you can't explore the depths of romantic passion without an occasional conflict or even fight, likewise you can't plumb the depths and riches of prayer unless you stand up to God. As the prophet Jeremiah discovered, God listens to our feisty words but we have to be prepared to receive his challenging words in response (cf. Jer 15:10-21). That is the nature of dialogue, whether on a human or divine plane.

St. Teresa captured in one spontaneous comment what other theologians have needed volumes to communicate. Job's wife expressed in one verse (cf. Job 2:9) what Job needed twenty chapters to convey. Although in Christian tradition, her response has been interpreted negatively, with St. Augustine labeling her "the helper of the devil", the Jewish interpretive tradition, generally more comfortable with lamentation, has been more sympathetic.

Perhaps Job's wife's prompting helped him to arrive at candor with God. Sometimes we need the example or coaxing of another in order to express ourselves candidly. Whether this is done positively or negatively depends on the person and circumstances.

> "It is obvious that pain, especially physical pain, is widespread in the animal world. But only the suffering human being knows that he is suffering and wonders why; and he suffers in a humanly speaking still deeper way if he does not find a satisfactory answer. This is a *difficult question*, just as is a question closely akin to it, the question of evil. Why does evil exist? Why is there evil in the world? When we put the question in this way, we are always, at least to a certain extent, asking a question about suffering too.
>
> Both questions are difficult, when an individual puts them to another individual, when people put them to other people, as also when man *puts them to God*. For man does not put this question to the world, even though it is from the world that suffering often comes to him, but he puts it to God as the Creator and Lord of the world. And it is well known that concerning this question there not only arise

> many frustrations and conflicts in the relations of man with God, but it also happens that people reach the point of actually *denying God.*
>
> For, whereas the existence of the world opens as it were the eyes of the human soul to the existence of God, to his wisdom, power and greatness, evil and suffering seem to obscure this image, sometimes in a radical way, especially in the daily drama of so many cases of undeserved suffering and of so many faults without proper punishment. So this circumstance shows—perhaps more than any other—the importance of *the question of the meaning of suffering;* it also shows how much care must be taken both in dealing with the question itself and with all possible answers to it.
>
> 10. Man can put this question to God with all the emotion of his heart and with his mind full of dismay and anxiety; and God expects the question and listens to it, as we see in the Revelation of the Old Testament. In the Book of Job the question has found its most vivid expression. (Pope John Paul II, *Salvifici Doloris,* "On the Christian Meaning of Human Suffering", 9, February 11, 1984).

Inspired by the feisty forthrightness of our female models, am I willing to give God a piece of my mind?

Do I believe not only that God desires such, but that I help myself and others at the same time?

When I have leveled with God, what was my experience?

Creative Life-Giving

There is no rational explanation for why God blesses some couples with children and prosperity but not others; it is a mystery of life and divine providence. However, those lacking such blessings can respond creatively and redemptively to this mystery by giving life in other ways. This doesn't eliminate the pain, but transforms it into compassion and tenderness. Reaching out to others takes the focus off ourselves and changes the orientation of our life. Instead of turning inward in response to the painful deprivation of children, we constructively direct our energies outward.

Many persons, myself included, owe much to celibate men and women. Sexually responsible single persons, nuns, priests, and brothers (celibate laypersons) support others (e.g., children, the disabled, the elderly, the poor) in so many ways. Many are living models of creative life-giving. Rather than focus their life-giving energies on a family, they spread it out.

Unfortunately many in society look down on those (e.g., persons who choose or accept celibacy as a way of life and couples with large families) who make significant sacrifices in exercising their life-giving vocation. If you exercise your vocation in a unique manner and follow your conscience you are likely to experience both interior and external resistance. It will be a struggle. However, the rewards of peace of mind in this life and eventual residency with God and fellow believers infinitely compensate for this.

Life-Giving is a Life-Long Lifestyle

A life-giving disposition is not constituted by a one-time choice or experience. Neither does it take away the pain of life's profound deprivations. Couples unable to bear children bear the scars all their lives. Other ways they give life become a salve which soothes and diverts their attention from the pain. The memories and wounds recede but remain. Even turning them over to God does not mean that they will not affect us. Paul himself was denied relief from a perplexing affliction, not because God wanted him to suffer, but because He wanted Paul to trust completely in God:

> "Therefore, to keep me from being too elated, a thorn was given me in the flesh, a messenger of Satan to torment me, to keep me from being too elated. Three times I appealed to the Lord about this, that it would leave me, but he said to me, "My grace is sufficient for you, for power is made perfect in weakness" (2 Cor 12:7-9).

We never really accept life's profound losses; at best we simply reconcile ourselves to them and find other outlets for our love and energies. The fact that procreation is a positive commandment uttered in a positive context can inspire individuals and couples to adopt a positive approach to whatever challenge they are given.

God has bestowed on us the creativity necessary for making the best of our situation. We can trust that He will provide the graces necessary for giving life according to His will and living with the results.

We should not draw a sharp distinction between procreation and other forms of life-giving. All of us need an ongoing dose of life-giving, both as giver and recipient.

Life is a continuum of relationships. We can view fertility in a more healthy, integrated manner if we link it with other forms of life-giving such as adoption, care for disadvantaged children and the elderly, and outreach to persons in need such as the homeless, the mentally ill, and the poor.

What are ways that you can give life within your present means and circumstances? What forms of outreach do you feel drawn to? What first steps can you take to share yourself and your gifts with others?

Bearing Children With Your Hearts: Giving Life in Other Ways

St. Augustine made the classic statement that parents who adopt a child bear them in their hearts. Throughout this book, and hopefully continuing in our lives, we will consider alternate ways of bearing fruit when preferred ways are barred. We will discover that God's power is strongest when we are weakest, and that we can cooperate creatively with God in redeeming our difficult situations. It is at the moment when we seem least capable of bearing fruit that we can do so astoundingly (cf. 1 Cor 1:26-31; 2 Cor 11:30).

A profound twentieth century example of perseverance bearing fruit posthumously is Charles de Foucauld. A missionary who received little support for his work and was murdered during a raid by marauders, de Foucauld's influence has grown in both spirituality circles and in the mission field. His life and death is testimony that appropriation of God's perspective on fertility and success can endure the grave, and transform unbearable situations into life-giving ones for those who come after us as well.

The Larger Picture of Fertility

It is not enough to reference biblical infertility passages or to draw insights and inspirations from life. These must be integrated to form a balanced perspective, one that transcends the prejudices and trends of the times and the impulses of the moment.

In the next chapter, we will reflect on the second half of the Bible's first commandment, that of exercising stewardship over creation and fulfilling our potential. We will discover interesting similarities between this and the vocation of procreation.

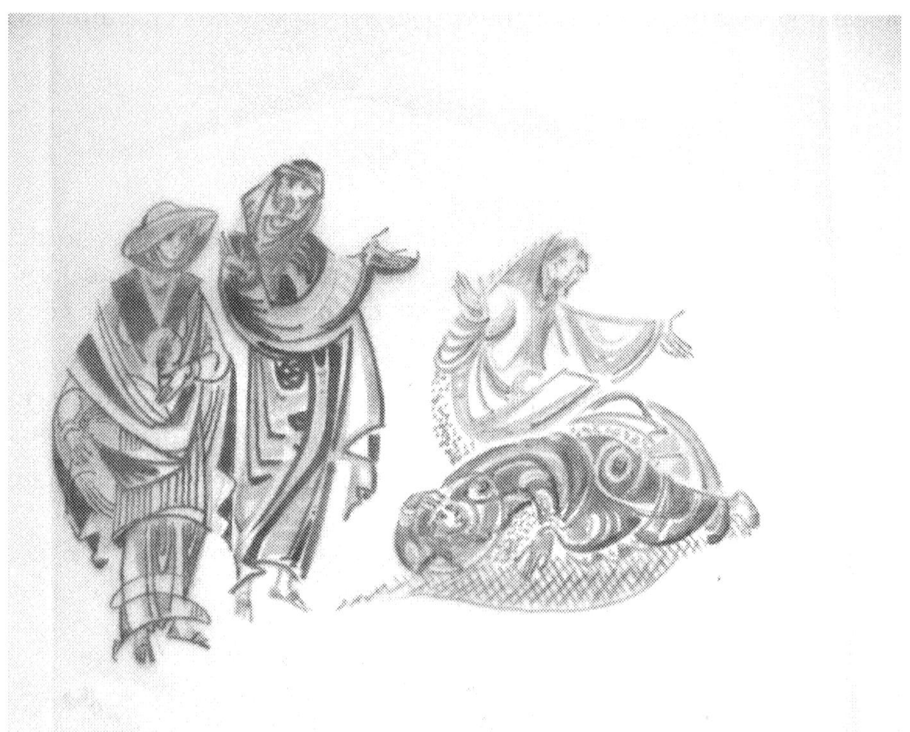

Figure 2. Ruth on the threshing floor.

Chapter two introduces the concept of functional (in)fertility and the metaphorical dimension of (in)fertility as presented in Scripture and as experienced in life. Ruth, Naomi, and Boaz illustrate this in their persistence amid difficult circumstances and their gracious helpfulness and hospitality. As discussed in the chapter, individuals and couples experiencing either biological or functional infertility can give life and be fertile metaphorically and functionally through their outreach to others, particularly those in need.

Chapter Two

Infertility as a Metaphor for Life's Limitations: Expanding our Definition

The Symbolic Dimension of Infertility

In the Bible and life, infertility is a symbol of frustration, impoverishment, and deprivation. Literally, it means an inability to bear fruit. Though its typical sense refers to procreation, it also figuratively applies to any thwarted endeavor or vocation.

The Bible uses this figurative sense in referring to God's involvement in human endeavors as opening or shutting the womb, that is, blessing or impeding human activities:

> "Shall I open the womb and not deliver? says the LORD; shall I, the one who delivers, shut the womb? says your God" (Isa 66:9).

The Bible, like us, refers to children as the fruit of the womb and success as bearing fruit:

> "Jacob became very angry with Rachel and said, "Am I in the place of God, who has withheld from you the fruit of the womb?" (Gen 30:2).

> "Sons are indeed a heritage from the LORD, the fruit of the womb a reward" (Ps 127:3).

> "Beware of false prophets, who come to you in sheep's clothing but inwardly are ravenous wolves. You will know them by their fruits. Are grapes gathered from thorns, or figs from thistles? In the same way, every good tree bears good fruit, but the bad tree bears bad fruit. A good tree cannot bear bad fruit, nor can a bad tree bear good

fruit. Every tree that does not bear good fruit is cut down and thrown into the fire. Thus you will know them by their fruits" (Mt 7:15-20).

"I am the true vine, and my Father is the vinegrower. He removes every branch in me that bears no fruit. Every branch that bears fruit he prunes to make it bear more fruit" (Jn 15:1-2).

"... as you bear fruit in every good work..." (Col 1:10)

"So it is with a woman who leaves her husband and presents him with an heir by another man.... Her children will not take root, and her branches will not bear fruit" (Sir 23:22, 25).

The Effects of Infertility

When couples desiring offspring are unable to procreate, they feel unfulfilled. The future looks less promising. Their views of God, themselves, and their spouse are affected. The procreative impulse has vast effects, particularly on women.

Infertile couples typically experience an aching emptiness. They might feel abandoned by God or their partner, or even blame themselves. Women often feel bad about themselves when they are the source of the infertility. They know that this feeling is irrational and they may nod their head when others tell them not to feel this way, but that doesn't diminish the power of the emotions.

One of the reasons this book is so imbued with biblical inspirations is that the Bible has a consoling and therapeutic authority that can penetrate our human defenses. Abbot Thomas Keating, O.C.S.O. has termed this healing of the conscious and subconscious mind "divine therapy."

If the root of the infertility lies with our partner, we are tempted to project our frustrations onto them and initiate a cycle of blaming and resentment. Then, minor frustrations take on disproportionate importance, and it becomes difficult to unpack our emotions and differences and determine what our real grievances are.

However, once we become aware of this development, if we remain disposed to work things out we can discuss our frustrations and begin to put things in perspective. A competent therapist can be of assistance in this unpacking endeavor. However, the key is to stop the cycle of negativity by emphasizing the positive within and between us, while gently but honestly addressing areas of conflict and immaturity.

Parallels Between Biological and Functional Infertility

People with traumatic losses undergo similar feelings and challenges. One of the ways we can put biological infertility in a healthy perspective is by seeing it in the context of other losses and deprivations:

Miscarriages, particularly when several occur

Death of a child

Premature death of a spouse, parents, or siblings

Disability of self or loved one(s)

Catastrophic losses or accidents

Unexpected job loss, financial reverses, or business failure, particularly amid heavy financial responsibilities

Prolonged unemployment or underemployment

Chronic financial difficulties

Prolonged loneliness

Discrimination that prevents you from utilizing your gifts and capitalizing on opportunities

Destruction of reputation

Intimate violations, whether of an emotional, social, physical, or sexual nature

Infidelity, betrayal, or abandonment by a loved one

Because of the subjectivity of human experience, it is difficult to speak precisely of the effects of a trauma or tragedy. The circumstances listed above have both unique and common aspects, including parallels to the experience of biological infertility.

For example, if a couple can't have children and their siblings are producing them seemingly effortlessly, they may feel left out and discriminated against by God. Why us? Likewise, if I am not able to find a tolerable, living-wage job, I may be envious of others with good positions.

Sometimes people presume that infertile couples do not want to have children and consequently make insensitive remarks that embarrass or offend. Likewise, when we encounter a difficulty that becomes public knowledge, we may feel singled out, labeled, and judged wrongly.

Single people who wish to find a partner but encounter a string of frustrating relationships can relate to partners who are unable to expand their relationship through children. Women who want to be mothers have something in common with persons who want to be a spouse. Each seeks intimacy and an outlet for their love, gifts, energies, and emotions.

Reflect on your experience of any of the above difficulties and consider their effect on you. Can you see any parallels between your situation and the experience of infertility? Consider deepening your understanding of both through reflection and sharing with others.

Solidarity in Suffering

Resolve is a national organization providing telephone counseling and up-to-date information on infertility. They have local support groups in many areas. Their website is resolve.org and their email address is info@resolve.org.

There are support groups for most wide-spread afflictions. You can usually find out if there is a local chapter by consulting your library or the internet.

A spirit of openness and empathy are more important in determining our ability to share with others than the details of our circumstances. Each person and circumstance is unique. Two persons undergoing the same affliction can manifest an entirely different response. We may have more in common with someone suffering from a different affliction than with someone who is experiencing similar difficulties. We can learn from both similarities and differences, and support each other through communication and pooling of resources and energies.

Expand Our Horizons

When we suffer from any significant affliction, the natural tendency is to turn our attention inward and be preoccupied with our problems. However, perhaps the most universally applicable therapy for coping with suffering is to reach out to others. Your attention will be diverted and you'll expose yourself to the positive energies and experiences associated with empathy and outreach. You'll often discover how good you have it, and that things could be far worse.

There is an old story that God invited all those unhappy with their burdens to place them on an altar and select burdens more to their liking. Everyone who took God up on His offer ended up selecting their own burdens.

What opportunities do I have for reaching out to others?

In what way could my/our situation be worse?

If I was given an opportunity to exchange burdens, would I?

Marvin's Multiple Maladies

Marvin was having difficulty getting over his divorce. He and his wife Maggie wanted children but were unable to conceive. Marvin thought that the infertility played a major role in the divorce, but Maggie emphasized other grievances. Unfortunately, her anger and his imprudent responses were such that they never got around to unpacking their complaints and determining what the fundamental problems were.

In any event, Marvin didn't want the divorce, and tried his best to achieve a reconciliation. Despite his efforts, his ex-wife became increasingly bitter towards him. He felt rejected, alone, and inadequate.

Like most divorced men, Marvin's support system was small and sporadic. He had only two confidants, and one was his minister. As the realities of the divorce took root, Marvin developed a low-grade form of depression. (Those suffering from persistent or severe depression may wish to consult a physician or counselor.)

Marvin quickly found that the answer to his problem was not another mate. He wasn't ready for a serious relationship, and had not gotten over his ex-wife. Marvin felt like he was in limbo; he wanted to move forward, but emotionally he wasn't ready.

Fortunately, Marvin disdained idleness, and was always looking for something to do. He channeled his energies positively by working with children at a local treatment facility. He developed a healthy attachment to the children, and looked forward to spending time with them.

It would be warm and fuzzy to report that Marvin met someone while volunteering at the facility, but such was not the case. He still experienced extensive bouts of loneliness and discouragement. However, Marvin kept himself so busy with work, volunteer efforts, and exercise that he didn't have time to dwell on his plight. He took one day at a time, and filled up his leisure time with hobbies, socializing, and cultural activities.

Marvin remained disappointed with life, his ex-wife, and himself, but that didn't stop him from living. He avoided serious illness while recovering from his trauma (such shocks make us more susceptible to sickness), and actually seemed in better spirits than during the latter days of his marriage, where he was constantly dealing with one upset or another. In reaching out to others, Marvin also got more in touch with himself. He developed a better understanding of his beliefs, wounds, strengths, and weaknesses.

There are many ways of exercising our maternal and paternal inclinations. Marvin shared his paternal energies and presence with children deprived of a father. In this way his suffering became redemptive, bringing healing to others and himself.

Jesus remarked "Those who find their life will lose it, and those who lose their life for my sake will find it" (Mt 10:39). Viktor Frankl, the Jewish psychiatrist and survivor of Auschwitz who founded logotherapy, a branch of psychology that emphasizes the importance of personal motivation and meaning, observed that we can bear most anything if we have a "why" or reason and can find meaning in our situation. Christians identify this as the redemptive dimension of suffering, which is rooted in Jesus' redemptive suffering, death, and resurrection.

In what ways can Marvin's situation or response be an inspiration to me?

What is my motivation for living life to the full? How can I put more energies into what inspires and rejuvenates me, and less into what depresses me?

The Mindset of Moving Forward

One of the keys to moving forward amid affliction is not looking back excessively and subjecting ourselves to an endless round of second-guessing. If only I had done this earlier... If only I had made this choice... If only, if only...

Such speculation serves no constructive purpose and is far from objective. It becomes an endless cycle that swallows us up and diverts us from what we *can* affect: the present. Hindsight is 20-20, but foresight is always blurry. As discussed in the last chapter, if we do our best and act sincerely, we can in good conscience accept the results and make the best of them.

Dwelling on the past can be a subtle crutch. We can distort and oversimplify it, and attach ourselves to its nostalgic aspects. Oh, how good things were. Oh, how free of anxieties we were. We can immerse ourselves in fragments of our past and thereby distort the whole. We selectively remember the past in accordance with our present disposition.

In moderation, reviving happy memories can be a healthy expression of sentimentality. Being inspired and consoled by nostalgia is normal, particularly when there isn't much to celebrate in our present. However, to avoid stagnation, this has to be combined with steps to improve our present.

Healing and growing is always a balancing act. Moving forward and letting go of absorption with the past is easier said than done. The past is an asset that should not be disposed of indiscriminately. Unless we learn from the past, we are likely to repeat it. And we can't learn from the past unless we reflect and dialogue on it. We need others' help particularly because we cannot be objective about our blind spots, weaknesses, and limitations. Experience is an effective teacher when absorbed in proper doses and in combination with the guidance and support of others.

If we spend time in reflection, prayer, and dialogue with competent confidants, counselors, and persons with similar afflictions we can identify the right time and way for moving forward. Otherwise our life is frozen experientially and we neglect the opportunities of the present.

Communicating with Absent Parties

In divorce or death situations, healing may be complicated by the fact that the person with whom we have either positive or negative memories is no longer with us. We cannot obtain their feedback or reassurance.

Since there are at least two sides to every story, it always helps to consider the opposite view point. We can simulate a therapeutic dialogue with our counterpart either through professional counseling, journaling, creative visualization, or prayer. We can write a letter to them, and then write back both how we think they'd respond and how we'd like them to respond.

We can write an imaginary conversation that enables us to express ourselves while placing in their mouths both what we think they'd say and what under optimal circumstances the best in them would say. This allows us to make allowances for their weaknesses in the spirit of Jesus' prayer on the cross: "Father, forgive them; for they do not know what they are doing" (Lk 23:34).

This constructive, concrete approach is better than going around and around in our head with recycled conversations and regrets.

This exercise and forum is non-confrontational and affords us an element of control. It can provide a measure of closure that enables us to move on with life while holding on to the positive memories.

Say we have lost a child. Or we never had one, but wanted one dearly. We can use our imagination to communicate with the child and share our sorrow. Through the grace of God and the natural process of releasing emotions, we can gain some sense of peace and reconciliation.

Of course, if at any point this exercise becomes too intense or painful, immediately desist and if necessary seek support from others.

With whom would I like to communicate? What would I and they say?

How do such communications affect me?

Facing the Present

Unless we address these unresolved issues, we will inflict new persons in our life with frequent references to our past, making them feel like an extra or bystander. Worse, we might act out these issues on them.

In summary, we shouldn't deny our past or neglect opportunities to learn from or build upon it, but neither should it be a crutch or substitute for courageously facing our present and future. A difficult period in my life illustrates this challenge.

During my mid to late thirties, I encountered a series of traumatic losses and setbacks. Though they were spaced out, their cumulative effect was significant.

I was full of doubt, confusion, and regret. Fortunately, I had two mentors who were supportive and wise. They helped me looked at things more objectively and avoid imprudent decisions and paths. They helped break my fall and encouraged me to get back up again.

When we are dealing with any trauma or tragedy, it is important to have competent guidance. We need empathetic and perceptive dialogue partners who are not simply yes-men. Those who validate our bitterness and self-pity and inflame our negativity do us a disservice.

Others can only help us so much. I spent just a few hours a month with my mentors, so I had to come up with the majority of coping responses on my own.

Therapeutic Exercise

One of my chief remedies was already in place: physical activity. Exercise was helpful for clearing my mind and exorcising some of my harsher thoughts and emotions. As the name implies, workouts can help us work out negative energies and put them in perspective.

One of my cardinal rules for exercising was not to put pressure on myself. I played organized basketball from grade school to college, and had enough of pushing myself to exhaustion. I was not equipped physically or mentally for such a disciplined regimen.

My primary form of exercise is swimming, and in twenty years of almost daily activity I have never counted laps or forced myself to swim at a certain pace. I don't even pressure myself to swim for a certain amount of time. I cease my workout when I feel like it, although I try to swim at least fifty minutes and do a small number of semi-sprints at the end. It is easier to sustain consistent exercise when you make it manageable and even enjoyable and avoid unnecessary pressures.

Positive Diversions

Anyone who works through a trauma or tragedy will tell you that work, exercise, travel, community service, or a hobby can be helpful for taking your mind off your problems. When we are engaged in constructive activity, we can't worry about or blame ourselves for things we can't control. However, each of these outlets must be kept in moderation; otherwise we will fail to develop other important aspects of life. I think by now you are seeing how essential balance and moderation are for coping with any affliction or obstacle. Extreme responses only create more problems.

Of course, not all afflicted persons or couples are able to concentrate on constructive activities and devote sufficient energies to them. When this is the case and your grief impedes all your activities, you need time and therapeutic help.

Fortunately, I had plenty of constructive activities to keep me occupied. For most people work is the most accessible diversionary tactic. It can channel our energies in a way that builds up ourselves and others.

My most productive writing periods have always been when I was coping with a major affliction or obstacle. I was focused and angry, and expressed my frustrations in a positive manner.

Of course, I still had to pursue other therapeutic activities such as those described below. I remembered the balance principle and made a point of not immersing myself in work so much that I became isolated, obsessed, and one-dimensional. Here again, I was blessed by nature and nurture because I am not by nature a workaholic.

I find St. Paul's words to be eminently true: "No testing has overtaken you that is not common to everyone. God is faithful, and he will not let you be tested beyond your strength, but with the testing he will also provide the way out so that you may be able to endure it" (1 Cor 10:13). God has allowed painful experiences to cross my path, but He has also given me activities, resources, and supportive relationships for coping with them.

Helpers

At this point a word in honor of "helpers" or support persons is in order. In the last chapter, we spoke of God as helper as a complement to human help. However, humans are God's primary instruments of support. Occasionally we should reflect on how others have helped us, and how we can help others.

There is no way I could have coped with my crisis if I had not had such a loving and balanced upbringing. As one example, if my mother and football coach had not persuaded me to stick out a difficult first season, I would probably not have developed the habit of perseverance. I was capable of writing this book only because I learned early in life to stick with a worthwhile project even when things were not going well. We usually know when we are in over our heads and it is time to move on to something else.

Who have been the key developmental influences in your life?

How might recollection and affirmation of their supportive efforts inspire you and them in your current crisis?

Coping Responses

Attention to hobbies, travel, and cultural activities kept me from overdoing work while at the same time taking my mind off my miseries. What better time to develop a hobby or cultural interest than when you are stressed and in need of a diversion?

I also took refuge in prayer, communing with nature, reflection on the Bible and other spiritual books, and journaling. This was invaluable in enabling me to work through my "infertile" period; that is, a time when life and my efforts were not bearing the fruit I desired.

I cannot speak highly enough of journaling. How much anguish I was able to get down on paper and out of my system. I learned many things about myself in the process of circumventing conscious and social filters by writing them down in confidence. I wrote how I felt, and discovered many emotions and insights that I would otherwise have missed. Journaling can function as a handy and portable counselor and sounding board, and an instant stress-reliever.

Prayer helped me calm down and tell God how I was feeling. Having unloaded my emotions on God, I was then able to sit quietly and listen. God's grace pierced my pride and false security, inspiring me to acknowledge my mistakes and weakness and to accept my dependence on God and others.

I experienced the consolation identified by St. Paul as "peace beyond understanding" (Phil 4:7). This is not a blissful feeling of well-being or an escape from reality. It is an inner calm and a deep sense of God's presence that braces you to face the day. It mitigates your impulses to exceed your boundaries and limitations. It helps you let go of tendencies to try to control what is beyond your province.

Bible reading was helpful in that it gave me inspired guidance and consolation. The Bible provided solid food for thought and criteria for living at a time where I had to make crucial decisions and undertake significant initiatives (e.g., moving, starting a new phase of my business, developing new friendships and business contacts).

One thing I did not do was inundate myself with trite and simplistic self-help books. In fact, I consciously avoided them. I knew that my situation was unique, and required a nuanced response that exceeded the scope of most self-help books. One reason I wrote this book was to fill this void.

I consulted professional and academic resources in areas in which I needed special help. These complemented the resources and activities mentioned above.

By engaging in an integrated combination of the above activities, I was able to work through a period during which I went over and over the past. Finally, with the help of prayer, good counsel, and the practical realization that life goes on, I was able to move on, though in truth the memories remained and the sadness lingered.

When our hurt is deep and unresolved, recycling it is an ongoing temptation. Fighting this only exacerbates its hold over us. We must find an offsetting constructive activity or purpose in life. Many of humanity's greatest advancements came from people responding redemptively to deep wounds.

Sometimes we have to go through the valley to make it to the peak, so we should forgive ourselves for occasionally getting stuck while licking our wounds. It's like we're wounded soldiers in a battlefield hospital, recovering from our debacle while gathering ourselves for the battle ahead.

Amid my dilemma, over-analysis bore little fruit because I didn't have sufficient data to arrive at an informed conclusion. Those who contributed negatively to my circumstances were not going to dialogue with me honestly and respectfully, so I could only arrive at their motivations by conjecture.

Human behavior retains an element of mystery, even to ourselves, so there is no point in trying to assign motives and rationales to persons who refuse to discuss them with us in part because they don't fully understand or accept themselves. How can they respectfully and effectively communicate with us when they aren't at peace with themselves? The best thing we can do is forgive them and ourselves, avoid bitterness, learn, and move on.

This letting go remedy applies particularly to biological infertility, where the source of our problem may be a mystery. The more compulsive pressure we put on ourselves, the more counter-productive our efforts.

A Realistic Perspective on Letting Go

I do not mean to make letting go seem like a simple undertaking. It is imprudent, insulting, and insensitive to tell people dealing with a tragedy or trauma not to worry about it or not to feel bad. People dealing with grief need a listening ear, a non-judgmental demeanor, and a caring presence. They need encouragement and compassionate candor. They need to know that you are there for them and that they are capable of coping with their difficulties.

Letting go is not the same as giving up. It means not banging our heads against impenetrable walls, but rather using our heads to circumvent them. The ideal is to encourage ourselves, or others when we are in a support position, to seek positive alternatives as an antidote to recycling and projecting negativity.

For example, if we are dealing with biological infertility, we can consult good books and other resources on the subject and implement our coping plan a step at a time. With confidence in ourselves and in God, we can find little ways of responding constructively. Eventually our efforts will bear fruit, though not necessarily in the way we envisioned.

With experience, reflection, and counsel, we can learn when to let go and when to hold on, and how to negotiate the thin line between responsibility and acceptance.

How do we achieve optimal efforts without trying too hard and slipping into counter-productive behavior? No book can answer that question, but you can. The principles and activities recommended in this and other chapters will help you arrive at the answers right for you.

Summary

Let us conclude with a review of attitudes and activities for coping with either biological or functional infertility. Throughout the book we oscillate between the two because of their common issues and the importance of seeing suffering as a continuum.

- Recognize the link and continuity between biological and functional infertility. This enables you to identify their related and cumulative effects in your life, and to relate more empathetically to other afflicted persons.
- When you are suffering, do not isolate yourself or engage in self-pity and over-analysis. Reaching out to others broadens your horizons and deepens your insights. Self-absorption isolates us from the therapeutic resources and consoling presence of others and the therapeutic effects of our own outreach.
- A fun and enriching way of expanding your horizons amid grief is to develop hobbies and personal interests. You become a more well-rounded person and give less energy and attention to worries and regrets.
- Release your tensions, clear your mind, and refresh your body and spirit by periodic exercise.
- Let work become a positive outlet for your energies. Difficult periods are often the setting for our most creative and substantive efforts, as we are rooted in the real world rather

than the ivory tower of abstract and isolated ideas. Consider your finest achievements, and the circumstances surrounding them.

- Though the topic is beyond the scope of this book, sufficient sleep and a healthy diet are essential to holding up well during difficult times. Amid our frenzied pace, such basics are easily overlooked. The consequences of addressing or ignoring these staples of health and well-being are significant.
- If so inclined, develop your spirituality through prayer, meditation, and spiritual reading, perhaps utilizing the *lectio divina* process discussed in the Introduction.
- Utilize a journal for communicating your thoughts and feelings in a safe context. You will get a first hand perspective on what is going on inside you.
- Exercise moderate access to happy memories from the past. When you sense it is time to move forward, find venues and forums for building new memories. Healing and growth occur by learning from the past, preparing for the future, and living in the present.
- Move beyond blaming, shaming, framing (projecting your issues onto others), and defaming (speaking harshly of others). You can't do anything about the past, and you can't be objective about your own or others' choices or behavior in hindsight. Be humble enough to accept your mistakes and correct them in the future. Make allowances for others and offer forgiveness, knowing you need such as well.

  Negativity towards yourself or others isn't going to solve anything. If others have offended you and refuse to address your pain, ask God to help you forgive them, one forgiving intention at a time, then leave them in God's hands. He alone can judge and remedy such situations.

  Usually there are mitigating factors in situations, things we have limited control over. You can't accurately recreate the past either mentally, emotionally, or spiritually. That was then, this is now. Do the requisite work to gain sufficient understanding of yourself and your circumstances, then move forward in a positive manner.

The best way to overcome seemingly insurmountable obstacles is to go around them by developing alternate strategies. Letting go doesn't mean letting up, but letting God guide you in your efforts by doing your best to discern His will and accept divine providence. In other words, not forcing or fighting things, but flowing with them. This doesn't mean avoiding all challenges or confrontations, but seeking compromise, conciliation, and integration when appropriate.

- Move forward in small steps. Don't try to work through everything at once. Set your sights on manageable improvements that build momentum and confidence. Change is best absorbed gently and gradually. Patience enables us to develop the coping strategy that works for us.

The didactic books of Proverbs, Ecclesiastes, and Sirach (one of the seven books included in the Catholic and Orthodox Old Testament but not in the Protestant or Jewish canons) contain an abundance of inspired counsel that can supplement the above and ground it in divine wisdom.

In this chapter we focused on universal attitudes and activities for coping with trauma and tragedy. Many of the insights and remedies discussed in later chapters are based on the values, principles, and activities discussed in this chapter.

In the next chapter, we will encounter one of history's most famous infertile couples, Sarah and Abraham, and draw parallels between their situation and ours.

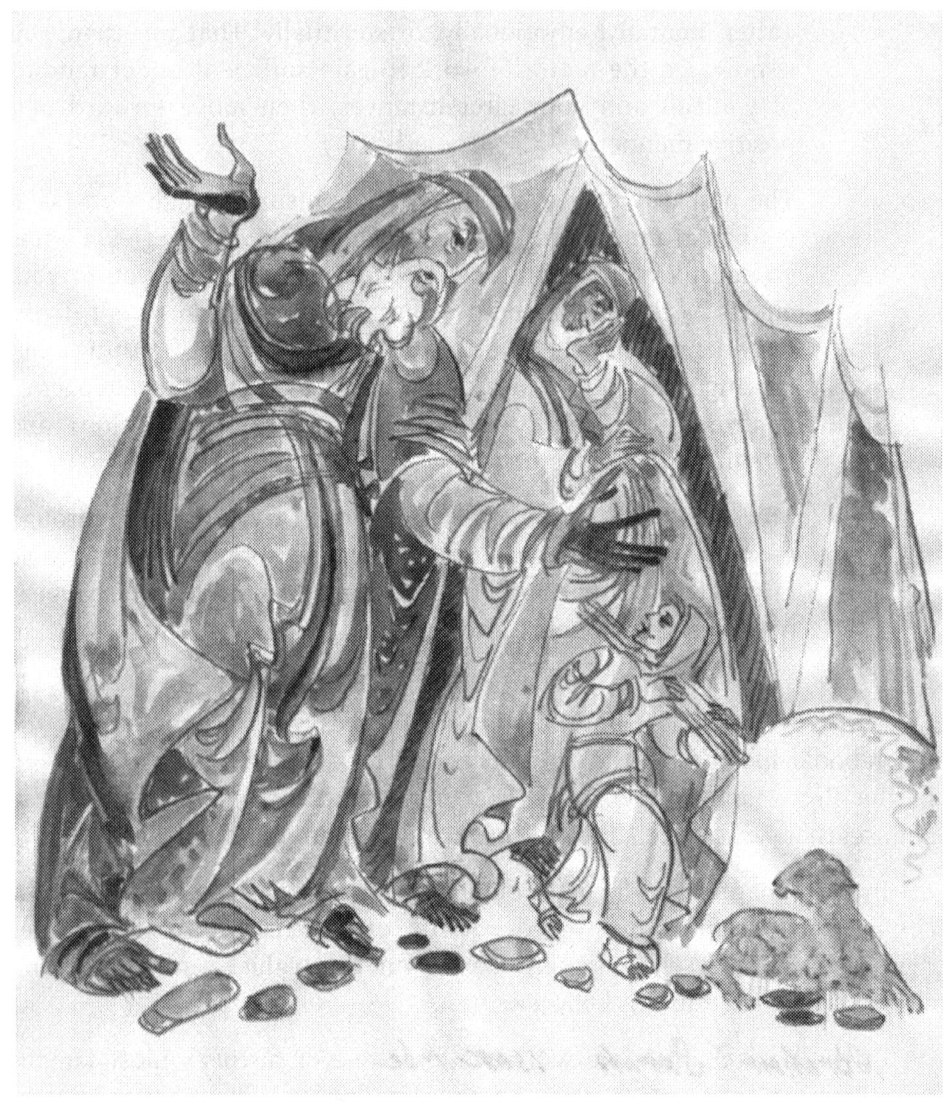

Figure 3. Sarah and Abraham.

Both Sarah and Abraham had become so resigned to their childlessness that they laughed at the divine prophecy that God would bless them with a child. Their sense of hopelessness was such that they wouldn't even put their trust in God's word. However, this didn't stop them from being hospitable to others, and giving life in other ways. According to their individual personalities and in ways representative of both gender tendencies and human nature (Sarah denied laughing when God questioned Abraham about her skepticism, and Abraham tried to convince God that they should settle for another choice for his heir), they persevered amid doubt. We can relate to them as models of imperfect faith who remained faithful to God amid vacillation, mistakes, and inner and interpersonal conflicts.

Chapter Three

Infertility and Hope

Strange Timing

You're an elderly shepherd in ancient Mesopotamia, the cradle of civilization, living a relatively comfortable life among loved ones, when all of a sudden God interrupts your tranquility and breaks into your life. He tells you to uproot yourself and your family and head for a foreign land where you will be vulnerable strangers. Leave your security for the insecurity of fidelity to God's word. You are given no blue print or travel plans, only an invitation and a promise.

Despite the fact that Sarah had reached menopause, Abraham and Sarah received a promise of posterity. They were going to bear the unbearable. Abraham and Sarah trusted in God's word, but like all of us, had their doubts.

Abraham was seventy-five when he received God's call. He was retirement age. God sure has funny timing. Why is it that He asks the improbable when we feel least capable of achieving it?

Have you ever felt that God put before you a challenge that was beyond your capabilities?

What experiences have you had of God's or life's bad timing? How did it affect you? How did or can you learn from it?

How is God asking you to bear the unbearable in the present?

What happens when you follow God's lead and pursue the improbable?

Holy Insecurity

Before and after Abraham, the holy people in the Bible lead insecure lives. If they're not running from kings (Moses, David, Elijah, Joseph and Mary) or being subjected to painful punishments (Joseph, Daniel, Jeremiah), they're getting grief from their own (Jacob, Moses, David, Amos, Jeremiah, Ezekiel, Paul). Little wonder that a destabilizing affliction like infertility becomes the opening symbol of the destiny of the Jewish people.

Such uncertainty goes against human nature. It's difficult to accept in any era, but particularly in our security-obsessed society.

The Bible describes Abraham's response to God's travel plans succinctly: "So Abraham went, as the Lord had told him" (Gen 12:4), accompanied by servants and his nephew Lot. Abraham's insecure journey starts out with little fanfare.

Likewise, when we undertake a positive endeavor or new direction in life, we usually do so accompanied by doubts, concerns, and limited resources, along with hope. However, God sees what is in our hearts and what others do not see. He doesn't always affirm us in a way that we can perceive right away. He didn't affirm Job to his face until the last chapter of the book (cf. Job 42:7, 9).

How is your life insecure? What parallels do you detect between Abraham's upheaval and your challenges? How might they make you a better person?

Risk as a Catalyst of Greatness and Fulfillment

Most of our greatest accomplishments are rooted in risk and faith. Any worthwhile undertaking is fraught with obstacles and uncertainty. To quote a maxim found in many cultures, "every beginning is difficult."

We have no guarantee of success or well-being when we embark upon an education, career, geographical move, or marriage. If we spend too much time considering the risks, we'll never take the first step.

Choosing to have children or pursue a significant project or goal places us in a vulnerable position. We are giving up control and comfort, and entering the unknown. This makes us susceptible to the sorrows and spices of life. We should affirm ourselves for trying. It would be easier never to accept the challenge and begin our journey.

Of course, doing nothing doesn't protect us from suffering. Bad things can happen anywhere and anytime. Excessive risk aversion invites one of the deepest forms of regret: the knowledge that we have wasted our gifts and opportunities. Each of us has a legacy of both realized and unfulfilled potential.

Have I affirmed myself and loved ones for setting out into the unknown? What can I do to reward good intentions and efforts?

In what areas have I become self-absorbed, complacent, and satisfied with mediocrity?

What can I do to shake myself out of my lethargy? What small steps can I take to utilize the gifts/resources and opportunities I have received?

That's Not In the Contract...

As happens in life, the unexpected occurs. Abraham's adopted homeland undergoes a famine, and he is forced to flee to Egypt. As an alien he has no rights, and with a beautiful wife he fears for his life. In order to protect himself, Abraham maneuvers and Sarah goes along with him. She poses as his sister, and eventually the lie is exposed to Pharaoh, who sends them away.

This is an example of the providential, pragmatic, and perilous dimensions of Abraham and Sarah's lives. They bend principles in order to survive, and God rescues them, but not before they have to sweat it out.

Can you relate to Abraham's pragmatism under fire? In what situations have you made compromises ostensibly in order to avoid a worse evil?

When you bring your situation and response to prayer and reflection, what do you discern are the moral considerations and the Holy Spirit's promptings?

When we embark on any vocation or significant endeavor, particularly when our objective is to be of service to God and others, we can expect the unexpected. A good friend's mother once told me that if we knew what the future would hold, we wouldn't want to go through with it. Who would want foreknowledge of difficulties? Who could bear up under such knowledge?

Only Jesus. His multiple predictions of his passion and death reveal another dimension of his incomparable suffering. His willingness to go through with his mission, epitomized most dramatically in the garden of Gethsemane and on the cross, is a sublime testament to his love for us.

The profound Epistle to the Hebrews explores the implications of Jesus' full and unrepeatable participation in and transformation of human suffering. We can read this along with 1 Peter, James, and St. Paul's most personal epistles, 2 Corinthians and Philemon, for encouragement amid trials.

Jesus, Peter, Paul, and all the martyrs and saints invite us to share in the Lord's sufferings, consolation, and redemptive mission (cf. 2 Cor 1:5; Col 1:24) through persevering acceptance of our own cross. The Gospel of Luke alone supplements Jesus' admonition to carry our cross with the modifier "daily." Luke underscores the personal aspect of our passionate relationship with Jesus by presenting the repentant thief on the cross as the only believer to call Jesus by his name, rather than "Lord", the more typical address in his Gospel (cf. Lk 23:42).

What crosses am I being asked to bear cheerfully and hopefully today?

Amid the daily living out of this vocation, how might I more fully access the support and consolation present in the Scriptures and the Christian community?

Perhaps no vocation contains such unexpected and gut-wrenching developments as marriage and parenthood. Your destiny is partially out of your hands. Many variables come into play as people and circumstances change.

The Clashing of Linda and Leo

Linda and Leo got married with many unexpressed expectations. Both thought that their marriage would be for life. Leo expected Linda to support him in all his significant endeavors. So far, she had.

Linda wanted a life of domesticity. She sought the tidy house and a handful of children, and did not mind leaving the workforce. She'd rather be home, as her mother was. Leo had gone through several jobs, but always worked. He barely made enough for them to live on.

Linda was into economic and social security, while Leo desired emotional and spiritual security. They never discussed these differences in detail during their engagement. Who wants to bring up such intense subjects? Doesn't love conquer all?

Within a year of their wedding, Leo lost his job and began his own business. At first, Linda was very supportive, helping him out whenever she could. She graciously and unpretentiously made heroic sacrifices that even Leo did not fully recognize or appreciate, to his eventual regret --- how easy it is to overlook the loving intentions and efforts of those closest to us. Her selflessness was particularly praiseworthy given the demands of her own job. Inspired by their vision of a successful business and their love for each other, they pulled together amid the difficulties of starting a business, and Linda never uttered a discouraging word.

All this time, Linda provided the primary means of financial support. Though she never said anything, she was anxious for Leo's business to start turning profits soon. Being the bread-winner wasn't her vision of marriage, particularly in the early years.

Linda's work hours suddenly increased, and she underwent more stringent supervision. This kept her away from home longer, and she began to develop resentment, first towards her employer, then in subtle, even unconscious ways, towards Leo. This wasn't what she bargained for from either. Since she couldn't do much about work, the natural target for her frustrations was Leo. How frequently we project our disappointments and failed expectations onto those closest to us who deep down usually want the best for us, but are not always able to communicate or actualize this in an appropriate fashion.

As their lives and relationship seemed to stall, Linda's parents became concerned. They liked Leo, but were not entirely comfortable with him.

Linda and Leo still got along, but there were more blow-ups and prolonged intensities. All this time, they had been trying to have a baby. Both felt ready and were hopeful.

After not conceiving despite several years of trying, they suspected that something was wrong. It was. Both had conditions making it improbable, though not impossible, for her to conceive. With Leo's business difficulties and their up and down relationship, adoption did not seem a viable option. Their relationship began a downhill turn. Only they could turn things around. Usually such turnarounds require the compassionate and competent support of loved ones, friends, peers, and therapeutic and pastoral professionals, which in real life is all too uncommon. This drama is repeated in so many people's lives, resulting in a variety of endings.

How might I address a current negative trend in my life or relationships?

Linda and Leo have come to you for counsel. What do you say to them? What remedies and suggestions do you offer? How do you break their problems into manageable components? How do you get them to recall and focus on their positives?

What implications do your responses have for similar challenges in your life?

The Ambiguity of Infertility

We don't know anything about Abraham and Sarah's relationship prior to God's call, nor do we know precisely how infertility affected their relationship. We can only imagine as to whether their relationship was smooth or rough.

As evidenced by their perseverance through tough times and Abraham's profound grief at Sarah's death, it seems they were compatible in their old age. However, there's no guarantee that they started that way. Through love, communication, commitment, and perseverance, many couples grow into compatibility, while others grow apart.

Abraham and Sarah's history is only partially revealed to us, but our history as individuals or a couple is readily accessible. How foolish we would be to ignore it.

Construct a timeline of your life individually or as a couple. List the significant and transitional events, the high, low, and pivotal points. How does your history shed light on your current circumstances?

The only biblical couples whose infertility-based conflicts are reported with any specificity are Jacob and Rachel (cf. Gen 30) and Elkanah and Hannah (cf. 1 Sam 1). Even then, not so much is said that we don't need to read between the lines and make inferences based on our perspective and experiences. The Bible leaves the texture of their relationship to us, inviting us to draw personal parallels, applications, and insights.

In both the Bible and life, each couple deals with their situation uniquely. There is not a one-size-fits-all solution to intimate problems. We need to seek our own solutions, to discover what works for us, and not feel bound to common practice or what the experts say.

Am I/we willing to look beyond popular opinion and trends and develop a customized solution to problems? In what way is my/our situation unique?

How have customized solutions worked for me/us in the past?

Impatiently Waiting on God

Abraham and Sarah's dilemma is no different than yours and mine. God takes His time in delivering on His promise. Have you ever known God or life to operate consistently according to your timetable and agenda?

What experiences do you have of God coming through, but only at the last minute or after you had given up on Him or the situation?

Naturally, Abraham and Sarah become impatient. The premise of a post-menopausal pregnancy was hard enough to take, and then nothing happens on that front while all kinds of unsettling events occur around them. When will God act? Could it be that they are being hung out to dry? We ask such questions when God delays in answering our prayers, or when disconcerting situations last for what seems an excessive amount of time.

We should not be surprised when doubts run deep. Even the saints have doubts. As discussed at the end of chapter one, God doesn't make it easy for those who come to him:

> "My child, do not regard lightly the discipline of the Lord, or lose heart when you are punished by him; for the Lord disciplines those whom he loves, and chastises every child whom he accepts.
>
> Endure trials for the sake of discipline. God is treating you as children; for what child is there whom a parent does not discipline? If you do not have that discipline in which all children share, then you are illegitimate and not his children. Moreover, we had human parents to discipline us, and we respected them. Should we not be even more willing to be subject to the Father of spirits and live? For they disciplined us for a short time as seemed best to them, but he disciplines us for our good, in order that we may share his holiness.
>
> Now, discipline always seems painful rather than pleasant at the time, but later it yields the peaceful fruit of righteousness to those who have been trained by it. Therefore lift your drooping hands and strengthen your weak knees, and make straight paths for your feet, so that what is lame may not be put out of joint, but rather be healed" (Heb 12:5-13; cf. Prov 3:11-12).

The Gospel of Luke reports that about an hour went by between Peter's second and third denials of Jesus (cf. Lk 22:54-61). What thoughts of abandonment must have gone through Peter's mind. Where were the other disciples? Why was Jesus letting all this happen? Was God really with Jesus?

Influenced by Old Testament images of God, Peter viewed Jesus as the deliverer, as one who triumphs and makes everything right. The fragility

Jesus displayed during the agony in the garden bore little resemblance to this image, and undoubtedly threw Peter into confusion. Were his hopes and dreams tragically misplaced?

Such vocational crises are among the most excruciating of trials, and can either diminish or strengthen faith. They can lead to despair, as with Judas, or they can make us compassionate and supportive of others in their trials, like Peter, the designated strengthener of the brethren (cf. Lk 22:31-34).

Have I experienced overwhelming identity confusion and vocational trials and doubts? How was I able to cope? In what ways did I grow?

Amid identity confusion and vocational obstacles, am I willing to be patient with myself as I struggle to be patient with God and others?

Affirmation from God

During a private moment with God, Abraham laments his childlessness, and God affirms that in time Abraham will have a natural son. Abraham believed God, and God took note: "And he believed the LORD; and the LORD reckoned it to him as righteousness" (Gen 15:6).

God responds to Abraham's obedience by making a covenant with him. By trusting that God will come through for us, we deepen our relationship with God. This is as important as the promise we are awaiting.

Few of us receive direct promises from God, as Abraham did. However, the Bible and the inspired literature of other faiths contain promises from God that, though general, can be counted on. Of course, only God knows when and how they will be fulfilled.

One of the most difficult aspects of faith is to trust in God when the concrete indications are that He has abandoned us. We don't have the direct dealings with God that Abraham and Sarah did. As Jesus said to Thomas:

> "Have you believed because you have seen me? Blessed are those who have not seen and yet have come to believe" (Jn 20:29).

Abraham and Sarah still had to weather perplexing events that put God's promise into question, so much so that they laughed at the prospect of its fulfillment. Their difficulties were such that God felt it necessary to affirm His promise to them (cf. Gen 15:1-6), and invite their trust and patience.

How God Speaks to Us

How does God affirm His promise to us in these post-biblical days? Primarily through prayer and contact with His word and initiative, found not only in the Bible but in creation and life events. If we persist in our dialogue with God, we will periodically experience intuitions or signs that God is present and faithful. (See discussion of the divine initiative in chapter one.)

Sometimes this will take the form of a biblical, mental, emotional, or experiential reminder of how God has come through for us either personally or collectively in the past. Sir 44-49 and Heb 11 are biblical litanies of God's dynamic activity in the life of Old Testament saints. They are an example of a collective remembrance that affirms our connectedness with believers of all eras.

God communicates with and affirms us through each other. We can likewise serve as God's ambassadors by building up each other with our words and deeds (cf. 2 Cor 5:20). This is particularly important when we are dealing with infertility or other afflictions.

We, and particularly couples, need to pick each other up amid trials. How difficult it is to support our loved ones when our positive feelings are offset by the resentments and hurts that accumulate with time and suffering. Praying and reflecting on biblical texts like God's affirmation of Abraham remind us of the importance of building each other up.

On what issues do I need affirmation? How might I communicate this to those I need it from?

Whom do I need to affirm? What are my obstacles to doing so? What small steps can I take to affirm others?

When Patience Runs Out

In Gen 16, the fireworks start. Sarah's patience is at an end, and she talks Abraham into having relations with her slave, Hagar. According to the custom of the time, the offspring would be considered Sarah's.

Gen 16:2 says that Abraham listened to the voice of Sarah. In Gen 3:17, Adam was reprimanded for listening to the voice of his wife. Scripture subtly affirms a woman's powerful influence over a husband who loves her. She can use this influence for good or evil. Just ask Samson (cf. Judg 16:4-31).

Hagar gets pregnant, and begins to look with contempt on her mistress. Feminine competition. Human nature. However, Sarah stills holds the upper hand, and she is not about to tolerate such arrogance. After blaming Abraham for the situation (a common projection between spouses), she gets his consent to have her way with the slave, who responds by running away. Sarah is a strong and persistent woman, and Abraham knows better than to stand in her way.

The Bible says only that Sarah dealt harshly with Hagar. Perhaps if it supplied the specifics, readers would be distracted by the injustice of Sarah's actions. Like Abraham, she was no angel.

Less than ideal behaviors and circumstances can be fit in, albeit awkwardly, to God's plan. Even when we respond inappropriately (especially to difficult, intense situations), God can still bring good out of it (cf. Rom 8:28). However, He prefers that we put as few obstacles in His way as possible. This also makes it easier for us.

In what ways have I responded to my difficulties in an immature and misguided fashion? Am I willing to accept responsibility for such, ask forgiveness of God and those involved, and move forward?

Do I believe that God can achieve His ends even when I fail to live up to my end of the bargain?

God Loves All Persons

God's providence does not extend exclusively to Abraham and Sarah. He steps in to help Hagar. He tells her to go back to her mistress and face the music, but with His protection. God doesn't like us to run away from problems. He is capable of helping us face our challenges.

God then makes a promise to Hagar similar to that given to Abraham. She will also have countless descendants. Her son's name, Ishmael, means "God hears." This is a fitting theme for persons dealing with any type of infertility. However, God's response may not be what we expect or desire.

You cannot put boundaries on God's love. He loves outside the lines. For the Jews, Hagar and her descendants, the Arabs, were outside the lines, but God loves them regardless. This unconditional love works in our favor, as we often stray outside the lines, whether we know it or not.

When I am outside the lines, do I think enough of God's love and providence to ask for His help?

Do I reach out to those outside the lines, or do I look down on them?

Gen 17-18 showcases Abraham and Sarah in simultaneously humorous and tense encounters with God. Both laugh to themselves when they are reminded of God's promise of a natural son. Abraham tries to persuade God to let Ishmael be his heir, thereby revealing his naiveté and shortsightedness. How does he think Sarah would feel about that? Has he forgotten her jealous streak and determination?

Gen 18 is one of the most profound chapters in the Bible. It has a particular relevance for persons struggling with severe afflictions or obstacles. Let's revisit the story.

Hospitality

Abraham is cooling off during a hot afternoon when unbeknownst to him he is visited by angels in the person of three guests. Being a generous man respectful of cultural values, Abraham views it as a privilege to extend hospitality.

Hospitality remains a cherished tradition in the Middle East. A stranger or traveler is vulnerable, particularly in an arid climate filled with contentious clans and countries. Human decency compels even adversaries to extend compassion and the necessities. Amid the aridity of biological or functional infertility and the resulting contentiousness we feel towards God and perhaps others, exercising hospitality is a way of transcending our situation and our negative inclinations and summoning the best in ourselves and the human spirit.

We should not pass over Abraham's hospitality lightly. The Epistle to the Hebrews cited his behavior as an inspirational example: "Do not neglect to show hospitality to strangers, for by doing that some have entertained angels without knowing it" (Heb 13:2).

Invoking Scripture's universal and existential dimension, we can infer that hospitality has an abundance of manifestations and implications, which can vary by person and situation, and we need not restrict personal applications to exact literal correspondence to the text. Likewise we should not think that the unwitting engagement of angels is also limited to its historical occurrence as recorded in the Scriptures. Jesus identifies all service to humanity as service to him (cf. Mt 25:31-46).

In his 1984 encyclical *Salvifici Doloris* ("On the Christian Meaning of Human Suffering"), Pope John Paul II asserted that Christ's identification of the so-called corporal works of mercy --- addressing the fundamental impoverishments of vulnerable persons such as hunger, thirst, loneliness, illness, and nakedness --- should be interpreted in a broad, inclusive sense, thereby encompassing all acts of charity.

Taking St. Paul at his word "Then each one will receive commendation from God" (1 Cor 4:5), I believe that couples or individuals dealing with any significant affliction or obstacle who reach out to others and do not give up on life or God will receive special commendation from God.

Compassion expressed through a mobile form of hospitality is a central value in the parable of the good Samaritan (cf. Lk 10:25-37), which was uttered in response to a question as to who constitutes our neighbor. The priest and Levite mistakenly put ritual observance above hospitality, while the religious outcast, the Samaritan, fulfilled the spirit of the law. He made the extra effort of putting the man up in an inn and offering to reimburse the innkeeper for any additional expenses on his way back. St. Paul ends most of his letters thanking others for their hospitality, and urging his communities to be hospitable to fellow missionaries.

Jesus was often the recipient of hospitality, and in both familiar (e.g., the home of Martha, Mary, and Lazarus) and unexpected quarters: from Zacchaeus, the hated tax collector (cf. Lk 19:1-10), and from the sinful woman whose dramatic anointing of Jesus serves as preparation for his burial (cf. Mk 14:3-9). The Bible notes that Zacchaeus was anxious and happy to welcome Jesus. Our welcoming of others, particularly the vulnerable whom Jesus identified himself with (cf. Mt 25:40), will not be overlooked:

> "Come, you that are blessed by my Father, inherit the kingdom prepared for you from the foundation of the world; for I was hungry and you gave me food, I was thirsty and you gave me something to drink, I was a stranger and you welcomed me..." (Mt 25:34-35).

> "Whoever welcomes you welcomes me, and whoever welcomes me welcomes the one who sent me. Whoever welcomes a prophet in the name of a prophet will receive a prophet's reward; and whoever welcomes a righteous person in the name of a righteous person will receive the reward of the righteous; and whoever gives even a cup of cold water to one of these little ones in the name of a disciple—truly I tell you, none of these will lose their reward" (Mt 10:38-40).

Being hospitable to others takes our mind off our problems and puts our energies and resources to good use.

Whom can I be hospitable to today?

Am I willing to accept the hospitality of others, particularly as I age or become dependent?

How might infertile couples be hospitable to others, beginning with themselves?

How might persons thwarted from fulfilling their potential extend hospitality to themselves and others?

Joint Hospitality

Abraham and Sarah work together to provide hospitality for their guests. They are a team. Throughout the Bible's lengthy description of their escapades (Gen 12-22), there is never a hint of oppression by either partner. Their individual power bases never become an obstacle to their unity. They are a model pair in many ways, and through prayer, reflection, and application their example can rub off on us.

When their guests predict that next year Sarah will have a son, eavesdropping Sarah laughs to herself. Abraham did the same thing in the previous chapter when God foretold the birth of his son. (Who wouldn't be skeptical, even incredulous?) They exemplify the tendency of close-knit couples to think and act similarly.

Many couples emulate Abraham and Sarah in opening their homes to others, including on a long-term basis. Such guests can include elderly parents, grown children with their family, aunts, uncles, siblings, and adopted or foster children. Every person (especially children) taken in is a sublime act:

> "Then he took a little child and put it among them; and taking it in his arms, he said to them, "Whoever welcomes one such child in my name welcomes me, and whoever welcomes me welcomes not me but the one who sent me" (Mk 9:36-37).

We can also open our homes to others on a daily or temporary basis. For example, welcoming friends or out of town guests. Such deeds benefit us not only in the next life. They soften our hearts, and in the case of infertile couples, help create a welcoming disposition and environment that invites God to bless them with children.

Singular Hospitality

Single people also extend hospitality. The story of Martha and Mary, which immediately follows the parable of the Good Samaritan, serves as a clarification of its emphasis on hospitality: "Now as they went on their way, he entered a certain village, where a woman named Martha welcomed him into her home" (Lk 10:38). We should not miss the emphasis of Martha's hospitality. This distinguishing trait of Martha is likewise noted by the Gospel of John (cf. Jn 12:2).

Martha becomes preoccupied with the details of serving, while Mary touches upon the root of hospitality, which is welcoming God through attentiveness to His word. We welcome God when we welcome the vulnerable (with whom He particularly identifies) and those who proclaim His word and carry out His work (cf. Mt 10:40-42).

There are many ways of showing hospitality and receptivity to both God and neighbor. It brings fertility/growth/fulfillment into your life and the lives of others. Hospitality is not just an individual or series of actions, but a disposition and lifestyle.

In what ways and circumstances can I be hospitable to a vulnerable person or someone doing good who needs support?

How are my afflictions or obstacles transformed by my hospitality?

Divine Tact

Sarah thought that she alone was privy to her skepticism regarding the prophecy of the birth of her son, but she failed to take God into account. According to the custom of the times, God goes through Abraham to address Sarah's skepticism. It makes for an interesting scene: God asks Abraham about Sarah's behavior despite the fact that she is right there. Perhaps He anticipated Sarah's embarrassment and fear, and mitigated it by using Abraham as a mediator.

As a humorous example of His intimate knowledge of human nature and marriage, God alters Sarah's response slightly in order to avoid a confrontation. In her skepticism over the prophesied birth of her son, Sarah had pointed out both her own and her husband's old age. When God brings Sarah's skepticism to Abraham's attention—asking about it respectfully so as not to intrude upon marital intimacy—God deftly omits

Sarah's remark about Abraham's age. Divine tact. God doesn't want to be in the middle of a marital spat.

When Sarah, like Eve (cf. Gen 3:13), fails to acknowledge her lack of faith, God calls her on it. As with Eve, he confronts her gently. God seems to have a soft spot for good-hearted women, as well as an awareness that it might be easier on all concerned if He tones down the confrontation. The Bible is intimately aware of the dynamics surrounding marriage and family life, including the power and volatility of human emotions.

With this and a similar incident discussed below (cf. Gen 18:1-15; 21:8-14) in mind, we can petition God to mediate our partnership difficulties. He may not do so as obviously as in Abraham and Sarah's case, but He can change our hearts, open our eyes, and give us strength and guidance.

Have I invited God's assistance in my relationship difficulties? Am I persistent in petitioning His support?

Do I have any perceptions of God's interventions (divine providence) or support in my relationship(s)? How might this inspire me in my present situation?

Feminine Tact

One of the admirable traits of women is their intuition as to what to leave out when dialoging on intense issues with their husband or romantic interest. Only when anger, fear, or other strong emotions enter the picture do they sometimes compromise their discretion. Sarah is obviously aware of Abraham's age and might comment on this to herself, but she was sensitive and respectful enough to spare his ego. She exemplifies the pivotal role a wife plays in marital harmony!

Men are fragile beings who can be thankful that nature has implanted in most wives an innate sense of their husband's vulnerability. Of course, as with any gift, this can also be misused.

Do I exercise sensitivity and tact with my partner's vulnerabilities?

When we attack each other's vulnerabilities, we can pray this passage and ask God for help in exercising more discretion, respect, and gentleness in the future.

Abraham's Dialogue with God

The triangular conversation in Gen 18 between God, Abraham, and Sarah is followed by an extended dialogue between God and Abraham. It involves God's outrage over the sins of Sodom and Gomorrah, and His plan to exact justice. Given their close relationship, God decides that He will confide this to Abraham.

It is interesting how God countenances Abraham's intervention in what is seemingly God's affair. Abraham bargains with God, something we are inclined to do when we suffer.

Abraham's bold intercession reminds us that we should not hesitate to persistently express to God our needs and concerns, even if it takes the form of bartering or bantering. We should not be afraid to speak candidly to Him, to share our expectations and frustrations. God is not a remote overlord, but someone who wishes to be intimately involved in our lives. He wants to be dialogue partners with us.

Am I willing to address God from the heart? Am I willing to emulate Abraham in expecting much from God? Will I communicate my concern or disappointment when things seem chaotic and purposeless?

A Dream Come True

Finally, after much preparation, a son is born to Abraham and Sarah. He is fittingly named Isaac, meaning "he laughs", thereby reminding his parents that they laughed at the prophecy of his birth, and that its fulfillment is an occasion for joy. Another way of interpreting this is that Isaac had a laugh on them all.

It is interesting that all of the spoken words recorded in the Bible with regard to Isaac's birth are attributed to Sarah. Sarah speaks while Abraham celebrates. Sarah has played an important but secondary role in the story until now. Motherhood puts the woman front and center.

Here We Go Again

Of course, the end of Sarah's infertility does not mean the end of problems. The excitement would just be beginning were not Abraham and Sarah so old. A potential sibling rivalry comes to Sarah's attention, and she demands that Abraham get rid of Hagar and Ishmael. Sarah is jealous and possessive, and driven by maternal instincts. Once again Abraham defers to Sarah. It may have been a patriarchal culture, but a strong woman knows how to stand on principle in any era.

Abraham feels caught in the middle between the determination of his wife and his great love for his son Ishmael. Abraham feels intimidated by Sarah, and like Joseph contemplating Mary's unexplained pregnancy (cf. Mt 1:18-20), arrives at wits end in trying to come up with an acceptable solution. Fortunately, God comes to the rescue and assures Abraham that he can satisfy Sarah's demand without guilt or regret. So Abraham packs supplies and leads the child and his mother away.

This is the second time Sarah has driven Hagar away. Again God comes to the rescue. In part, the story of His intervention is an explanation of the origins of the Arabs, Israel's ancient neighbors. However, the main point is that God's providence is not exclusive to Israel, a theme that will resurface in the story of Jonah, this time with the dreaded Ninevites, known throughout the ancient world for their depravity and cruelty.

Given all that Abraham and Sarah went through to have him, Sarah's over-protective attitude is hardly surprising. Perhaps this and the traumatic adolescent experience discussed below caused Isaac to be inhibited in his social development. He is much less of a central and dynamic figure in the Bible than his father, sons, and grandsons.

God's initiative in our lives does not sweep away all our problems. Even Isaac, the promised son, experienced negative effects from the mysterious way providence and life played out. Later Old Testament figures likewise endured perplexing situations as part of God's plan. Hosea was commanded to stand by an unfaithful wife, Ezekiel lost his wife and took it extremely hard, and Jeremiah was forbidden from marrying.

When we experience the negative consequences of our heavy burdens, we should not presume that God is punishing us, nor expect to understand His methods. We can view ourselves in a long line of good folks whose experience of God's initiative is bittersweet. That is why it is important to freely express our frustrations to God and to hold on to our hopes that eventually, whether in this life or the next, God will make right what certainly isn't now.

Abraham and Sarah's dream came true, but I may be awaiting mine. Will I dialogue with God about my hopes, and tell Him of my disappointment and frustrations? Will I ask for the strength and wisdom to cope with my time of waiting? Will I wrestle with God, if necessary?

The Sheer Humanity of the Biblical Stories

Sarah is one of the most human characters in the Bible. I can imagine her carping at Abraham about Hagar first, and then Ishmael. She is not about to give way on a matter so close to her heart, maternity. The Bible doesn't specify how long Sarah had been complaining, but my guess is that like Delilah with Samson ("Finally, after she had nagged him with her words day after day, and pestered him, he was tired to death. So he told her his whole secret..." Judg 16:16), she wore him out.

Consider the great love Sarah had for Isaac. She sheltered him, and insisted on making things just right. She didn't wait all this time for nothing.

The Bible does not relate stories of otherworldly people who are inaccessible to us. It profiles flesh and blood characters with strengths and weaknesses like you and me. When we read the Bible we can insert ourselves into the story and discover parallels in our life. As pointed out by Carlo M. Martini, S.J., in the German foreword to *Through Moses to Jesus* (Ave Maria Press):

"In the history of Moses, as in the other events recorded in the Bible, we find realities that are repeated in the life of every individual. Anyone who is inwardly open and acquainted with prayer can find in the words of scripture what is needed for his or her life.

It seems to me that the decisive questions to be asked by each person are

* What does this scripture passage mean to me?

* What is it saying to me?

* How is it related to my life?

We might at first say, "It doesn't have anything to do with my life." But rather than remain with such a first impression, we should look for the cause and ask, "Why is there no connection between this Bible passage and my life? What would I want the connection to be?"

In this way, even a negative first impression can be a means of contact between what the Bible says and what we experience. Often this contact does not take place immediately, but only after we have entered into a dialogue, a wrestling with the words of scripture. Only then does it begin to shed light.

Such a dialogue is a decisive help toward prayer, which springs from our center and expresses our deepest yearnings. This is the aim of spiritual guidance: To help us express ourselves in prayer as we are, in keeping with our situation and nature.

Real prayer is not child's play. Scripture teaches us that prayer is a struggle, a battle. It places us face to face with our greatest difficulties. In prayer we are trained to look at the problems of our life with an open eye and to accept them, for human beings are often afraid to confront themselves."

Abraham's Test

Gen 22:1-19 is one of the most compelling stories in literature. It involves God's request that Abraham sacrifice his son Isaac, a repugnant prospect for the Israelites. The Old Testament frequently condemns infant sacrifice, which was practiced by Israel's neighbors. Only rarely did Israel's leaders engage in child sacrifice (cf. Judg 11:29-40; 2 Kings 21:6). How could God make Abraham and Sarah wait so long for a child and then renege on His promise, especially in such an unconscionable manner?

Double Trouble

The story of Abraham's test builds on previously introduced motifs. The saga of Abraham and Sarah is full of doublets or similar stories told in different ways. For example, twice Sarah is disguised as Abraham's sister (cf. Gen 12:10-20; 20:1-18). The second time, the theme of infertility and God's involvement with it reappears.

In punishment for King Abimelech's taking of Sarah (in Jewish tradition, Sarah is regarded as one of history's most beautiful women), God closes the womb of his wife and their female servants (cf. Gen 20:17-18). The infertility theme resurfaces. Abraham intercedes for them in a manner similar to Job (cf. Job 42:7, 9), and the women become pregnant.

When we hear these ancient stories, we should bear in mind that the Jewish people did not distinguish between primary (God) and secondary (natural causes, free will) causes. God was seen as the ultimate cause of everything. The classic expression of this is Isa 45:5-7:

> "I am the LORD, and there is no other; besides me there is no god. I arm you, though you do not know me, so that they may know, from the rising of the sun and from the west, that there is no one besides me; I am the LORD, and there is no other. I form light and create darkness, I make weal and create woe; I the LORD do all these things."

We should bear this theological distinction in mind as we contemplate God's unconscionable testing of Abraham.

Abraham's journey with Isaac comes on the heels of his journey with Ishmael. Imagine having to give up two sons as part of the fulfillment of God's promise. This is clear indication that when we submit to participation in God's plan, we let go of control and subject ourselves to perplexing and painful events that foreshadow joy and fulfillment.

Have I undergone experiences with similar conflicts or personal messages? What did I learn from them?

Sarah's Mysterious Absence

The drama of God's mysterious request unfolds in masterful fashion. The key figure missing is Sarah. Where was she when this instruction was given to Abraham? We have seen throughout their saga that God conducted most of His interventions and communications through Abraham. However, on something this critical, it is puzzling that Sarah is not informed.

Perhaps the most obvious explanation is that Sarah would not have abided the test. God works through humans as they are, and Sarah was hardly an ideal candidate for such a mission. God witnessed her jealousy and possessiveness on several occasions, and could surmise that she would be unwilling to let go of her pride and joy. What mother would abide such a test? Abraham likely recognized this and did not inform Sarah of God's command.

How horrible it must have been to receive so gruesome a command from someone you had grown to trust and respect. Also, Abraham had no one with whom he could confide and share his anguish. He was alone in his pain and confusion.

God gives no rationale when testing human beings. He simply invites obedience and perseverance and promises deliverance: "No testing has overtaken you that is not common to everyone. God is faithful, and he will not let you be tested beyond your strength, but with the testing he will also provide the way out so that you may be able to endure it" (1 Cor 10:13).

The Bible is silent with regards to Abraham's feelings, as it typically is in traumatic situations. It invites the reader to supply the feelings, based on their own experience. In this way the Bible draws us in and makes us realize that we are the characters, and that the story is also about us.

Have you ever felt that God has acted out of character or contradicted Himself by abandoning you or putting you in an unconscionable situation?

Why do you think God acts this way or lets such disastrous situations develop?

If we thank God when good things happen to us, can we lament His seeming inaction when bad things occur?

The Cathartic Question

The story supplies pertinent details and moves at a crisp pace, as if to camouflage the interior struggle undergone by Abraham. Everything comes to a head with an innocent question posed by Isaac: ""Father!" "The fire and the wood are here, but where is the lamb for a burnt offering?" (Gen 22:7)

Isaac unknowingly poses the question that should not be asked, the inopportune communication that brings to the fore the emotional and spiritual turbulence that has been festering, and potentially ignites it. Similar questions ring in our hearts when we are confronted with profound traumas and deprivations. God, everything is in place except the necessities.

Where are you? Why haven't you come through with the goods? Why have you let the situation develop in this manner? Why undermine my efforts and the mission You have given me? Why tease and test me this way?

We can imagine the confusion and anger stewing inside Abraham. It has come to this, and I have no answers. God's promise looks empty now.

Such gut-wrenching questions arise any time we are confronted with a tragic situation with no discernible way out. We don't know how to respond, except to proceed with grief in our hearts, mechanically putting one foot in front of the other. When will God intercede? When will the nightmare end? When will a resolution occur?

Modern examples of painful probes include when infertile couples are asked thoughtless, intrusive, questions by others, or when they experience pressure or derogatory comments from family members. These also occur when couples become insensitive to each other and say things better left unsaid. Often this occurs unintentionally, but the pain lingers nonetheless.

We know the ending to the story. Abraham is about to sacrifice his son when a voice from heaven calls "Abraham, Abraham", telling him to stop. This double call is rare in the Bible, occurring only six other times (Gen 46:2; Exod 3:4; 1 Sam 3:3-10; Lk 10:41; 22:31; Acts 9:3). It always signals a significant event and personal encounter.

The lesson is that God deals with us intimately and personally, particularly when the communication is of a challenging nature. God is not an arbitrary, whimsical deity who manipulates humans like pieces of a puzzle. He has a tender concern for His children, even as He puts them to the test. God knows what we are made of, but He wills that we find out first hand, and learn and grow in the process.

The story's happy ending continues, as Abraham spies a nearby ram which he substitutes as a holocaust. God almost got Abraham's goat, and now he got His.

Testing as an Invitation to Trust

Traditionally, interpretations (particularly the classic New Testament commentary in Heb 11:17-19) of this mysterious passage have focused on Abraham's faith. However, what also stands out is God's mysterious request. How could God ask this of a faithful believer? How could He allow a beloved to undergo such an ordeal? How could He pretend to rescind a promise long affirmed and anticipated? God's behavior seems as capricious as the pagans' deities.

One of the historical interpretations of this passage is that it reminded the Jewish people that God does not want infant sacrifice, which many of

Israel's neighbors practiced. Archaeological excavations have yielded evidence of sacrificial altars in the area mentioned in the passage, though the precise location of Moriah (cf. Gen 22:2) is uncertain.

The story also strikes at the heart of biblical faith, which means to trust completely in God, even to the point of giving up all you have, including your most prized possessions or relationships. Abraham gives us hope that though we compromise our principles along the way and encounter numerous doubts and difficulties, we can still work towards obedience and trust.

Avoiding bitterness amid infertility or other afflictions is a way of giving of ourselves and surrendering to God. We trust that He not only knows what He is doing, but will help us cope and bring good from our situation.

In which situations have I fought off resentment and bitterness and chose to make the best of things, even when I did not understand the purpose of my affliction? How might I build on this in dealing with my current affliction?

The Goal of Commitment

It is very difficult to remain faithful to God when you feel He has abandoned you, particularly when it involves a trauma with respect to a (potential) family member. God doesn't deny the difficulty of the challenge, but He still wants us to put Him first. Jesus was extremely demanding, and consequently lost many disciples:

> "Because of this many of his disciples turned back and no longer went about with him. So Jesus asked the twelve, "Do you also wish to go away?" (Jn 6:66-67).

The challenges of infertility and potential fulfillment converge in the total commitment demanded by Jesus in the following citation:

> "Whoever loves father or mother more than me is not worthy of me; and whoever loves son or daughter more than me is not worthy of

> me; and whoever does not take up the cross and follow me is not worthy of me. Those who find their life will lose it, and those who lose their life for my sake will find it" (Mt 10:37-39).

Jesus wants to be first in our hearts, even when we cannot bring life into the world or develop ourselves optimally and live the kind of life we desire. The spousal relationship, a frequent Old and New Testament symbol for God's relationship with His people, is perhaps the best way to understand this. A spouse wants to be first with their partner no matter what. They don't want to be second to anyone or anything. That is why difficulties arise when children are prioritized over, rather than alongside, the marital relationship.

Ways of Letting Go

Since we are using the Bible to help us understand the spiritual underpinnings of fertility and potential fulfillment, it is necessary that we take into account the entire message of the Bible, which is extraordinarily challenging. As indicated by Jesus in the last verse quoted above, when we let go of all of our inordinate attachments, even to life itself, is when we truly come alive.

An example of such letting go is the infertile couple that goes through the grieving process and then redirects their procreative efforts towards adopting a child or reaching out in another way. Another example would be the person who can't get a living wage job using his or her talents, but who does not become bitter and cynical. Or the rejected person who moves on with their life rather than nursing a vendetta.

Consider what happens in such situations. The infertile couple find others who need their love desperately. Were these individuals not to get it from the couple, they might not get it at all. The un\underemployed person becomes more in touch in reality, more appreciative of the essential things in life and the true value of money and work, and more compassionate towards others.

I have known a number of persons with good paying jobs who unhesitatingly spouted the corporate and capitalist creed, having little sympathy for persons unable to attain living wage employment. When the market forces worked against them and they lost their job, they either came to realize the narrowness of their former perspective or they became embittered.

The divorced person who does not gossip or retaliate not only avoids toxic feelings, but frees and prepares themselves for future relationships. If you treat an ex-spouse with dignity, you give an indication that you will likely treat a future spouse with dignity, and thus are more likely to attract dignified persons.

None of the persons discussed above or the many more suffering individuals that we could consider would choose their plight. Even with their positive attitude and actions, their circumstances remain far from ideal, and their sorrow remains. Who knows whether in this life they will reap in practical and material terms the good that they have sown. However, they are trying to love God even more than their potential children, fulfillment, and spouse, and they have Jesus' promise that they will eventually find their life.

In another passage (cf. Mk 10:28-31), Jesus promises that those who do not let human attachments impede their following of him will receive a hundredfold reward in this life as a prelude to heaven. This passage is also found in the Gospels of Matthew and Luke (cf. Mt 19:16-30; Lk 18:18-30), but only the Gospel of Mark includes the addendum "with persecutions." All of us are familiar with the sorrows and external resistance that accompany the joys of life-giving.

Have you ever had to let go of a loved one without preparation and perhaps prematurely or tragically? How were you able to retain your faith in God?

With regard to such experiences, are there things left unsaid that you would like to share with God or others, including perhaps in your journal or a letter to them?

What experiences have you had of persevering with God even when He takes away what you do not want to let go of? How has it affected you?

Be Like God: The Ultimate in Procreative and Potential Fulfillment

> "You shall be holy, for I the Lord your God am holy" (Lev 19:2).
>
> "Be perfect, therefore, as your heavenly Father is perfect" (Mt 5:48).
>
> "Be merciful, just as your Father is merciful" (Lk 6:36).
>
> Instead, as he who called you is holy, be holy yourselves in all your conduct; for it is written, "You shall be holy, for I am holy" (1 Pt 1:15-16).

The above citations show how confident God is in us, and how much He wants us to fulfill our potential. The way to do so is by mirroring God, in whose image we are created. Jesus came to earth to show us what God is like: "whoever has seen me has seen the Father" (Jn 14:9).

When we try to procreate, we share in God's live-giving capacity. When we reach out to others compassionately, we emulate God, who describes Himself as compassionate (cf. Exod 22:27). When we try to do the right thing, no matter the circumstances, we imitate Him.

Even when circumstances and the fruits of our labors are not as we would like, we should not assume that we are not fulfilling our mission and potential. To the contrary, being obedient to God by persevering amid obstacles is the height of potential fulfillment, for anyone can achieve and believe during good times.

God's Example

God does not ask anything of us that He is unwilling to do Himself. In offering up Jesus, God went through this test Himself. With Jesus, however, the sword was not halted, the damage not mitigated.

Who among us has experienced the misunderstanding, rejection, betrayal, desertion, abandonment, and persecution undergone by Jesus?

The answer is all of us, but not with the intensity and gravity that accompanied Jesus' suffering. God the Father did not spare Jesus from the pains of life; rather, He subjected him to them fully, though with a redemptive purpose.

Though Jesus has undergone the most brutal of tests as part of God's mysterious plan for the salvation of the human race, we are not spared of such possibilities. We also are asked to give up things dear to us. We encounter God's mysterious tendency to give us gifts, only to ask for them back. We have to undergo events that seem meaningless and irredeemably evil.

Surviving Our Test of Character

What God asks of Abraham and of us is to not cling too tightly to our hopes and dreams, but rather to subjugate them to God's will. In the end, God will come through, but in His way and time.

In the meantime, we may be filled with doubts about His methods and motives. We may wonder why He would permit our experience of infertility or whatever affliction we are undergoing. The story of the binding of Isaac, as the story is traditionally known in Judaism, reminds us that God does not expect us to understand His ways, but He does want us to abide by them. This is for our own good, however difficult it may be to understand and accept.

The Bible's unflinching description of God's preposterous request of Abraham is a candid recognition of life's and religion's contradictions, and invites us to view them from a faith perspective. Each of us must come up with our own interpretation, questions, and source of meaning, as complete answers are beyond our grasp.

I view God's unconscionable tests as His catalyzing our potential by inviting us to work towards unconditional faith, hope, and love. As with Abraham, he needs our trust and consent.

In what tests do I see seeds of growth?

What previous tests have made me a better person?

What happens when I pray my frustrations regarding God's tests? What happens inside me when, like Abraham seeking justice, I dialogue with God?

God's Free Gift

Our focus is on the relationship of Abraham's trial to that of individuals and couples dealing with various forms of infertility. This brings us back to the theme developed in chapter one. Fertility and potential are a gift. We are not owed posterity or prosperity. This is a hard pill to swallow, but ultimately we belong to God. We are clay in the hands of the potter (cf. Rom 9:20-21). Everything is gift (cf. 1 Cor 4:7).

This rubs against our individualism, but God is not running a democracy. Thankfully, God is supremely benevolent, and we can be sure He has our best interests in mind. However, as illustrated throughout the Bible, beginning in Gen 3-4, the companion of free will is suffering, and neither the Father nor Jesus has insulated us from this. To the contrary, just as the Spirit drove Jesus into the desert to undergo testing (cf. Mk 1:12), so our following of Jesus and the movement of the Spirit will likewise lead us to painful challenges. They invite us to join our sufferings with Jesus' and participate in the world's salvation:

> "I am now rejoicing in my sufferings for your sake, and in my flesh I am completing what is lacking in Christ's afflictions for the sake of his body, that is, the church" (Col 1:24).

From a spiritual and humane standpoint, what could fulfill our potential more than this?

The Dual Meaning of Suffering

This verse and the parable of the sheep and goats (Mt 25:31-46) are two of the most important and profound New Testament statements on the meaning of suffering. They are a staple of Christian theological reflections on suffering, and capture the dual meaning of suffering: to do good by our suffering (the redemptive aspect) and to do good to those who suffer (the compassionate aspect).

The Bible Mirrors Life

It is interesting that the Bible does not record Isaac having subsequent dialogue with Abraham after his poignant question discussed above. No mention is made of Sarah's reaction to the event, nor of any further words exchanged between her and Abraham. On some level, the traumatic test leads to an experience of isolation. Ultimately, we have to face suffering and death alone.

Perhaps understanding that Abraham did what he had to do, but still unable to cope with the prospects of her son's sacrifice, Sarah may well have curtailed communications, an experience intimately familiar to individuals and couples who suffer traumatic events. She dies shortly thereafter, and Abraham's mourning is described in detail, thereby attesting to his love for her and her significance in God's plan of salvation (cf. Gen 23).

It is interesting that Sarah dies before witnessing Isaac's marriage, while Abraham remarries. How true to life. So often good parents die before seeing their children grow up, and never experience grandchildren. Further, men whose spouse dies after a long marriage often enter into a second marriage quickly, particularly widowers with young children or divorced men with custody of their children. Generally speaking, in modern times men are less self-sufficient than women. These circumstances and more come within the circumference of the Bible's timeless expositions of and reflections on life.

Reading Between the Lines

I have taken considerable liberties in reading between the lines of Abraham's and Sarah's saga. Obviously they are partly a projection of my perspective and experiences. You are free to disagree and substitute your own insights.

Because the Bible often is sparing with details on its most significant events, we need to reflect both on what is reported and what is missing. Why did the author relate this detail, while leaving others to our imagination? Further, what does this mean in relation to our lives? The challenge in reading the story of Abraham and Sarah, as with the other stories in the Bible, is to make them ours, to discover ourselves in them.

Let us conclude with some synthesizing reflection questions. These can help us get closer to God, ourselves, others, and the biblical characters. In the next chapter, we will encounter an even more volatile infertile couple, Jacob and Rachel.

Do I see any parallels between Abraham and Sarah's relationship and my relationship(s)?

Do I feel comfortable dialoging candidly with God in the manner of Abraham (cf. Gen 18:16-33)?

Do I feel that God has pulled the rug out from under me in the sense of giving me hopes and expectations then letting them be dashed? Do I feel that God has reneged on His promises to me, and forsaken the efforts and relationships that I have cultivated in good faith?

Do I feel that God asks too much of me at times? When I feel like this, how do I respond? Do I share my feelings with God, or do I manifest my frustrations in a destructive manner?

Why do you think God seems to open doors for us, and apparently fulfill our dreams, only to permit a sudden reversal? Is it providence, life, or some combination? How have you reacted to such circumstances? How might you grow in response?

Why do you think Sarah was not consulted during Abraham's test? What is the significance then and now (to you)?

Put yourself in Sarah's place. How might she or you have reacted to post factum knowledge of the test? Do you think Abraham ever told her? If he did, how might that have affected their relationship? How would it affect yours?

How might Abraham's test have changed his relationship with God, Isaac, and Sarah? How have similar tests affected your relationship with God and others?

Imagine yourself as Isaac. Have you ever felt in the middle of a terrible situation, a true victim of circumstance? How did you cope and grow from it? Do you have related wounds that require healing? Perhaps you can conduct an imaginary dialogue with Isaac, as if he were in a support group with you.

Enter into Abraham's dilemma. How do you feel when God asks what you do not want to give? When you bring your confusion and frustration to God, how does God seem to respond to you? What do you sense, feel, or intuit?

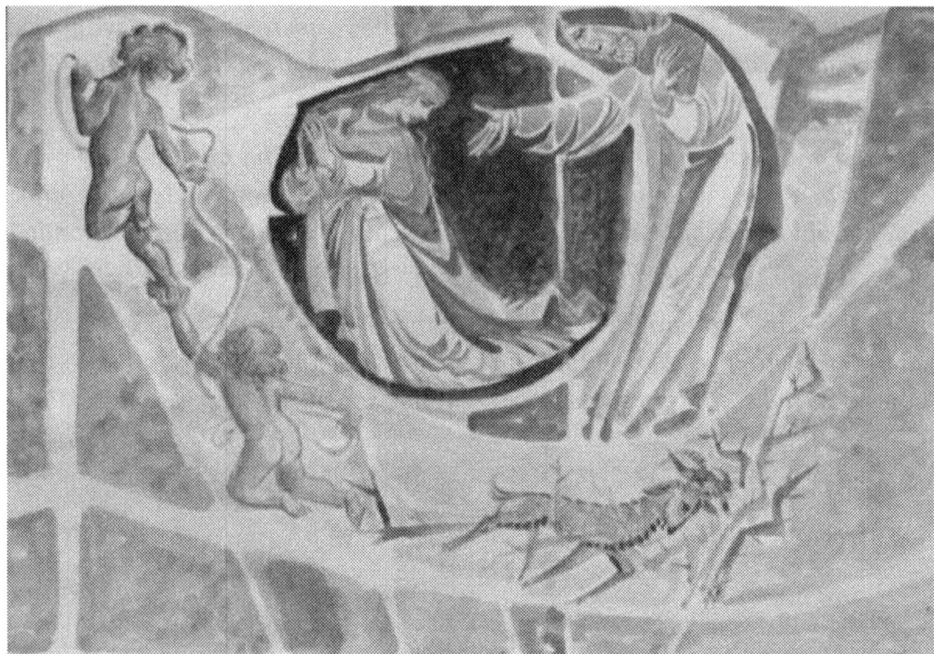

Figure 4. Isaac and Rebekah

The struggle between Isaac's sons began when they were in their mother's womb. Isaac petitioned God to make his barren wife fruitful. Be careful what you pray for. In the words of Jesus, "You do not know what you are asking" (Mt 20:22). It is important to persist in prayer, but we have to be ready to accept the consequences. I have no doubt that despite the heartache that ensued from their children's rivalry, like any childless couple, Isaac and Rebecca would bear it all again for their children.

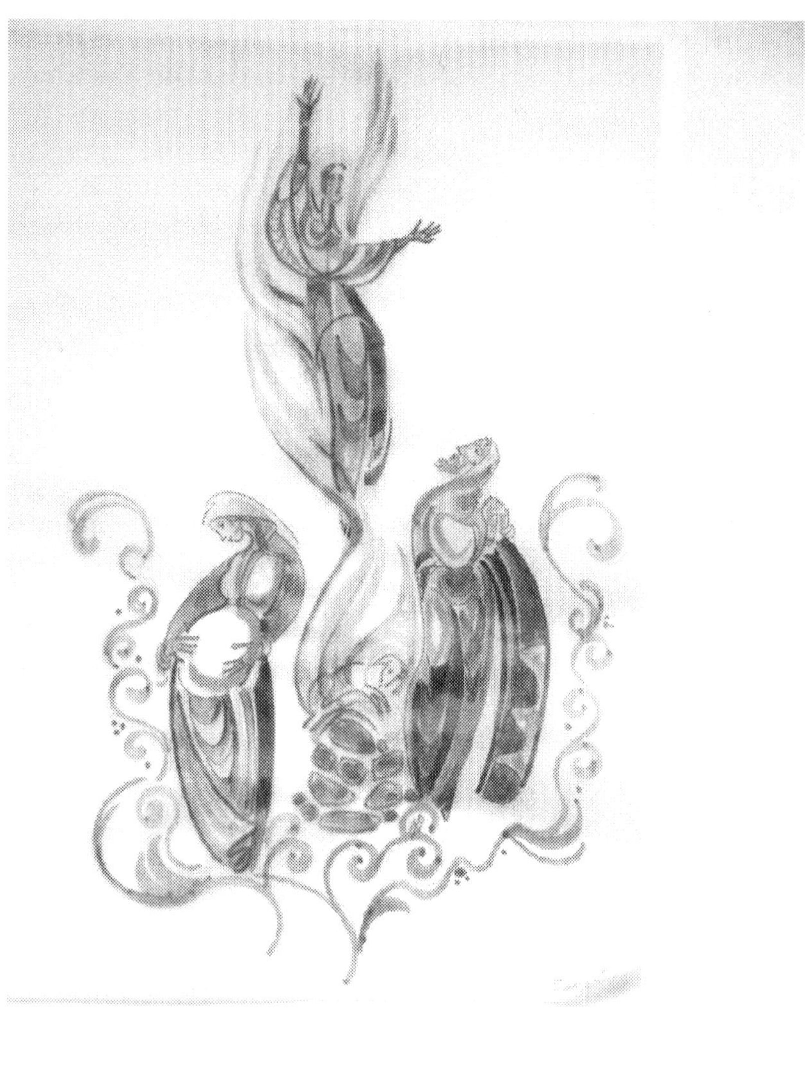

Figure 5. Samson's parents, who were greeted by the angel.

The infertility story of Samson's parents is instructional and unique in several ways. First, whereas in the Old Testament God and the divine messenger generally speak to a man, in this case the woman is twice visited by the angel. Second, she consults her husband both times in a deferential, respectful manner, and he in turn acts lovingly towards her and seeks what is in her best interests. When they discuss their encounter with the angel later, the anonymous mother of Samson correctly discerns that their encounter with God will not lead to their demise, as was expected in the Old Testament, for, with the exception of Moses, no one can encounter God and live. Like Abraham and Isaac before him, Manoa petitions God for guidance, and accepts it both from the divine messenger and his insightful wife. How pleasant and fruitful marriage can be when it is devoid of egotism and contentiousness.

The mother goes unnamed, but not unnoticed. She is an inspiration and model of humility, wisdom, and fidelity for persons, and particularly women, of all eras.

Chapter Four

Mixed Blessings: God's Bittersweet Answers to Prayers

While the Bible took several chapters to describe Abraham's and Sarah's struggle with infertility, it spends only one verse on Isaac's and Rebekah's situation:

"Isaac prayed to the LORD for his wife, because she was barren; and the LORD granted his prayer, and his wife Rebekah conceived" (Gen 25:21).

The biblical writers may have figured that they had covered much of the infertility ground while describing Abraham's and Sarah's saga, and Isaac is a more passive, less compelling character. His story may not have been interesting enough to support such detail. However, we can work with even this single verse and find applications to our situation.

Isaac didn't get married until he was forty, which was ancient for that culture. Given his traumatic near-death experience (cf. Gen 22) and his mother's protectiveness, we might infer that he was sheltered, scarred, and cautious, thus the long wait. Part of the fun and learning associated with the Bible is reading between the lines and using common sense and experience to make reasonable inferences.

Mixed Blessings

While Rebekah's pregnancy would seem to be cause for joy, it transpired with such pain that she despaired of life itself:

"The children struggled together within her; and she said, "If it is to be this way, why do I live?" (Gen 25:22).

Many women experience similarly traumatic pregnancies, even to the point of death. Life is full of mixed blessings. We get breakthrough, life-changing opportunities only to have them snatched from us before we can enjoy them fully. We form relationships only to have them fall apart despite the best of intentions.

For example, an engaged couple's dream bursts due to the death of one of the partners. A woman conceives after a long period of infertility, undergoes a difficult pregnancy, then has a miscarriage. An underpaid person works long hours for years at subsistence wages, then finally gets a promotion, only to have down-sizings eliminate the position shortly thereafter. A woman struggles to gain her due in a predominantly male profession, only to be undercut by her fellow workers, some of whom she considered friends.

When Job's blessings became mixed, and he began to lose the many gifts God gave him, he initially articulated the pious motto that has been recalled by many persons amid their experience of grief:

> "Naked I came from my mother's womb, and naked shall I return there; the LORD gave, and the LORD has taken away; blessed be the name of the LORD" (Job 1:21).

Job amazes us with his seeming acceptance, but soon his emotions erupt and he no longer can maintain such outward serenity. The tragedies and injustices of life wear down the patience of most persons, evoking outrage and a plea for relief.

Some people have the faith and temperament to trust God amid traumatic suffering. This itself is a gift, and they have their struggles and weaknesses in other areas. Most of us cannot operate like this; we cannot echo Job's words when life becomes calamitous. We need to vent our feelings and express our displeasure to God and others.

The book of Job was written in part to legitimize these feelings within a faith context and to inspire a deeper encounter with God through the sharing of these feelings. Job and his wife lose all their children and wealth, and Job loses his health, so there are direct connections to our theme.

The intensity with which Rebekah's twins struggle creates violent energies surging within her. Although like Job's wife she only utters one line (women can say a lot with a little, particularly in the Bible where they don't get their say to the same extent men do), we can infer that underlying it are a whole gamut of emotions to which we can relate.

Am I like Job's wife, who loses her patience with God and her husband when hope seems gone, or like Job, who manifests external piety despite inner conflicts? Whichever applies, how might I improve my response?

Job's conflict was with his wife and friends, while Rebekah's was with her children. In which relationships are your energies and emotions most aroused?

God's Mysterious Ways

Once again, we are witnessing God's strange methods. First, in the story of Abraham and Sarah, he delays fulfilling a promise and then feigns rescinding it. Then he answers the prayers of Abraham's son with a difficult pregnancy which almost leads his wife to despair.

These stories are comforting in the sense that they reflect life and shed light on our confusion and discouragement. We often experience responses to prayers and diligent efforts that initially seem delightful, but soon turn disturbing. Be careful what you ask for. God's answering Isaac's prayer is a fruitful topic for reflection because prayer is what humans often turn to amid troubled times, yet our experience of God's response and our own internal reaction varies greatly.

Have I experienced answers to prayers that delighted at first and then disturbed greatly? How did this affect me? What did I learn from it?

How can you grow as a person and in relationship with God when He provides such mixed blessings?

Seeking the Good of Others

When we read of Isaac's prayer being answered, we almost miss one of the most important elements. He prayed for his wife. He interceded for her. Isaac loved his wife so much that her happiness was as important to him as his own.

In our cynical age we are tempted to laugh at this notion and call it outmoded romanticism. Who can take such selflessness seriously? It contradicts the self-interest that permeates most modern relationship books. It is as if we believe reality can only be negative. If we open our eyes and hearts we will discover all around us, particularly in the mire of human brokenness and tragedy, examples of such selflessness. Children comforting parents and trying to help them during troubled times. Adult children reaching out to parents and grandparents, taking care of them in ways they were once taken care of. Grandparents putting their interests and activities on hold in order to help their children and grandchildren. These things don't happen just in fairy tales and old movies. They occur in our midst, if only we will take notice.

Disgruntled persons often vilify their former peers, partners, or someone who has hurt them. They are so blinded by emotions that they are unable to respond rationally and compassionately to rejection or failed expectations. Understanding and forgiveness are absent.

However, not all folks succumb to such rage. Some persons are mature, objective, and good-hearted enough to respond rationally and empathetically and extend the benefit of the doubt. They experience difficult emotions, but try to work through them through prayer, reflection, journaling, and counsel, rather than act them out.

For example, not every divorce or child custody arrangement is a battle. Some people find a way to civility even in unfortunate circumstances. It's not easy for them, and they make mistakes along the way, but their overall demeanor is caring and responsible.

The same is true of persons burned by economic injustices such as greed-driven down-sizings, hostile take-overs (particularly by corporate raiders unconcerned as to the effect on their actions on employees and the community), and executive irresponsibility. While others become bitter and project their rage onto the next person, they give their situation to God and cope with life as it is. Such acceptance often comes at a significant cost. In discussing one of the psalms of lament (where the psalm writer complains to God about his situation), Carlo M. Martini, S.J. points out that virtue and prayer do not shield us from suffering:

> "We should not think that those under persecution or suffering for the sake of the Gospel, for love of justice or liberty, live in a state of enthusiasm and euphoria. Often indeed they live under a tremendous burden of loneliness and fear, crying out to God without ceasing."[1]

When we find God's response to our prayers to be bittersweet, we can take consolation in the experience of Isaac and Rebekah. All the trying experiences they underwent did not occur independent of God's watchful care. These events, like those in our life, transpired in the context of God's benevolent providence. We'd like His plan to run smoothly for us, but that's not how it typically goes. If true love never runs smooth, then how can we expect our relationship with God to be free of strife?

What mixed blessings am I currently experiencing?

How has my experience of God's providence/initiative been bittersweet, a combination of sorrow and joy?

How have I responded to these ups and downs? How might I respond in a better way?

The Anonymous Birth of Samson

Judg 13:2-25 recounts the mysterious birth of Samson as foretold by an angel. This recalls the prophetic appearance of an angel to Abraham and Sarah. Samson's birth occurred during a difficult time in Jewish history, when they were subject to their enemies, the Philistines.

One of the interesting things about the story of Samson's birth is the anonymity of his parents, and in particular, his unnamed mother. It seems fitting to ask: why does God often call on obscure people to do His will? Why does this obscurity extend in this circumstance to the woman's name not being given?

---

[1] Martini, Carlo, M. *What am I that You care for me?: Praying with the Psalms.* (The Liturgical Press, Collegeville, MN: 1990, 36).

God Reads the Heart

God gives the answer to the first question numerous times in the Bible: humans judge by appearance, but God reads the heart (cf. Lk 16:15). God summons people to participate in an extraordinary way in His plan based on divine criteria rather than human standards and agenda.

Actually, God invites all persons to participate in His plan in an extraordinary way. However, we may not know it is extraordinary at the time, nor should we care. Living according to our conscience and trying to do what we think is right is the service God seeks. The Bible offers this definition of sin: "Anyone, then, who knows the right thing to do and fails to do it, commits sin" (Jas 4:17).

Consider Samson's parents. They had not been blessed by children, and the Bible says nothing of how this affected them. As discussed in previous chapters, this is so that we can fill in their response based on our experience, and thereby participate in the story.

We can contrast their experience of God's intervention with Isaac's and Rebekah's painful experience. The Bible does not mention Samson's parents' undergoing any agony as part of the pregnancy process. However, his mother is ordered by the angel to avoid alcohol and unclean foods (according to the legal prescriptions outlined primarily in the book of Leviticus), to not cut the boy's hair, and to dedicate him to God.

It is interesting that when angels appear to humans in the Bible, they rarely give complete instructions. They evoke questions as to how these wondrous deeds are going to occur. We can refer to it as divine intrigue. God gives us information on a need-to-know basis. He tests our faith for the purpose of deepening it and seeks creative cooperation rather than mechanical obedience.

Have you ever embarked on a mission or project with scant information, just enough to get you started? What did you learn from the experience?

Do you believe that God provides partial signs and pointers so as to test our fidelity and perseverance? What has been your experience of the way God works in this regard?

Can you discern God's presence and assistance amid your experience of biological or functional infertility? Can you perceive His subtle guidance and affirmations, as well as His mysterious allowing of disturbing situations which evoke feelings of disillusionment and abandonment, but also can lead to growth and healing?

Divine Symbolism

Like Isaac before him, Samson's father, Manoah, has his prayers answered. He wants guidance and asks for another divine intervention. He receives it, but in an unexpected way.

Once again the angel appears to Manoah's wife. This time she runs to get him, and he gets his chance to encounter God's messenger. Actually, Manoah receives no more information than his wife originally received, but at least he gets confirmation.

It is interesting that when Manoah asks the angel's name he declines to reveal it, pointing out that it is too wonderful. This recalls God's refusal to reveal his name to Moses at Mt. Sinai (cf. Exod 3:13-15). We might then ask why Manoah's mother's name is not revealed, and if this is a manifestation of sexism.

I believe that we would be well-advised to avoid assigning a sexist label to this story. First, the possibility exists that by the time this story was written down, the mother's name was lost. Second, the symbolism of anonymity may carry a universal message. There is another prominent example in the Bible of important persons not having their proper names reported. In the Gospel of John, Mary and John are referred to simply as the mother of Jesus and the disciple whom Jesus loved.

I believe we can see in Samson's anonymous mother a universal symbol of motherhood. God pays attention to her, and in His eyes her barrenness is no cause for shame. Rather, it is the seed of God's activity not only in the life of this couple and their son, but in the life of Israel as a whole.

We should note that Manoah's lineage (tribe) is reported by the Bible, but we are given no indication that he is a prominent person. He is a positive model of masculinity in that he believes his wife even when she tells him something extraordinary, he provides prudent leadership by seeking further guidance, and he expresses his gratefulness to God and the angel according to the religious understanding of the time.

How have your parents influenced your understanding of motherhood and fatherhood?

What other models of parenthood have been influential in your life?

The Risks and Uncertainty of Faith

As mentioned above, God typically conveys information on an as-you-go, need-to-know, basis. Jesus invites us to pray for our daily bread (cf. Mt 6:11), and to not worry about tomorrow (cf. Mt 6:34). God's initiative in our lives doesn't eliminate the need for faith and trust, nor does it provide immunity from difficulties. When you try to cooperate with God's involvement in your life, you are more likely to experience challenges and difficulties, through which God molds you into a more loving and mature person. Such growth usually has a painful dimension. God's blessings are mixed now in preparation for fullness in the next life.

For example, if they lived long enough, Samson's parents undoubtedly would have experienced much pain and anxiety over his exploits, some in fulfillment of God's will and some driven by his own agenda. His motives are mixed, as is often the case with us. To live and love fully is to be vulnerable to others, particularly loved ones. The alternative is a guarded, overly secure life that fails to satisfy and leads to stagnation.

Consider how infertile couples go about their lives in darkness, not knowing whether God will bless them with a child or not. Consider the abandoned spouse who still loves the one who rejected or betrayed them, and finds it difficult to move forward. They experience God's consolation and reassurance through the Bible and prayer, but their pain and challenge remains in one form or another. All they can do is take one step and day at a time.

Consider the unemployed individual who prays for divine help and periodically seems to get it in the form of promising job leads, only to find most of them are dead ends. While they learn in the process, it comes at a high emotional and financial cost.

Do you have any experience of God entering your life in a consoling but cryptic and confusing way? In what circumstances has He pointed you towards a direction or decision, then left you to make your way as best you can, while continuing to seek His guidance?

What have you learned, and how have you grown from such experiences?

Bearing the Fruits of Hospitality

In chapter 3, we discussed the essential role of hospitality in coping with biological or functional infertility. It is important to reach out to others even when we don't feel like it. That is when it is most meaningful.

Elisha was an influential prophet known for performing miracles. 2 Kings 4 relates the story of a wealthy Gentile woman who extended hospitality to Elisha whenever he passed through the area. Eventually Elisha inquired as to what could be done for her in return. Elisha's inquiry was indirect and triangular in a way that reminds us of Abraham's dialogue with God about Sarah in Gen 18. Also, when the couple's lack of a son is pointed out, the husband is referred to as old, just as Abraham was by Sarah.

In the widow's presence, Elisha directs his servant to ask what can be done for her, and selflessly she seeks no personal favors. She does not even mention that she and her husband have yet to bear a son, an heir to carry on the family name. She simply identifies with her people and avoids any request for personal gain.

In this way she reminds us of Solomon, who when granted a wish by God chose his people's interests rather than his own (cf. 1 Kings 3:5-15). After she leaves their presence, Elisha's servant speaks up for her and points out her plight to Elisha.

Anonymous Heroes

Many assuming people undergo terrible trials for which they ask little sympathy or support. These anonymous heroes, like the unnamed Gentile woman who cared for Elisha, often receive help only when their plight is observed by others. In contrast, others draw attention to themselves for the most insignificant and self-serving of reasons.

Widowed parents often find that after the mourning period for their spouse is over, there is no one around to help them. Some divorced persons face the many adjustments of single life without a supportive family or circle of friends. An unemployed person is left to rely on the cold and meager assistance of the government, while their gainfully employed friends lend little support.

Can I relate to Elisha's wealthy benefactor? In what ways have I gone about my difficult experiences in an uncomplaining fashion, doing what I need to do rather than making life miserable for others?

The Need for an Advocate

Sadly, not all anonymous heroes and heroines have someone speak up for them in a timely manner. So many people are without advocates. The rewards received by the wealthy Gentile woman are not experienced by many good-hearted persons.

This is where we have to bring creativity, common sense, and humble confidence to our reading of the Bible. A given story can only convey one circumstance, whereas in life there are many variations. The ending of the Gospel of John points this out: "But there are also many other things that Jesus did; if every one of them were written down, I suppose that the world itself could not contain the books that would be written" (Jn 21:25).

We can enter into dialogue with the biblical author, characters, and God, and share the details of our story. Inspired by the original story, we can transpose its essential values, principles, and challenges to our story and circumstances. We do this not to justify ourselves or to use against others, but to (re)discover that God is as active in our life as He was in the biblical characters' --- that our experience of God may not be as transparent or spectacular makes it no less significant.

If we are one of those persons who has few advocates, whom God seems to overlook, we need to speak up for ourselves and tell God of our needs. We need to persistently implore His help (cf. Lk 18:1-8) rather than act as a martyr.

The wealthy Gentile woman is unusual in the Bible in her reticence to ask for a favor. The Psalms and Gospels and Acts of the Apostles are filled with grieving persons asking for relief. Books such as Jeremiah, Lamentations, and Job contain some of literature's most eloquent and emotional petitions for relief.

Am I willing to speak up for myself to God and others, and ask for help?

When I have done this in the past, what has been my experience?

Am I willing to risk rejection and an exacerbated sense of abandonment when asking for help, and persevere even when God and others do not hearken to my plea? How am I affected when my cry goes unheard: "From the city the dying groan, and the throat of the wounded cries for help; yet God pays no attention to their prayer" (Job 24:12)?

Hopeless Resignation

When Elisha's servant predicts the birth of a son for the Gentile woman, like Sarah she hesitates to believe. She had gotten accustomed to her situation and the accompanying grief, and was perhaps a little hardened by it. She would be wary of having false hopes rekindle her latent anguish.

Many of us who have experienced biological or functional infertility have come to a similar point of resignation. We've lost hope of fulfilling our dreams, and have learned to live with our situation, albeit not as we would like.

In such situations we have to guard against cynicism, mediocrity, and despair. We have to avoid compromising our integrity and our zest for living. We have to believe that God will make things right, if not in this life, then in the next. We would rather not have to exercise such patience, but that is one of the virtues necessary for spiritual and psychological maturity.

False Hope

How often false hope becomes our tormentor! St. Augustine commented that two things kill the soul, despair and false hope. Infertile couples observe signs that they may have conceived, only to discover that their perception was mistaken. Families and friends hoping for the recuperation of a loved one see them experience an improvement followed by an unexpected decline that leads to permanent disability or death. A graduate saddled with loans discovers few employment opportunities. We move to another location to start a new life only to find that old problems follow and are joined by new ones. We devote years of life to our romantic partner in the belief that they share our commitment, only to have them walk out on us on a moment's notice.

False hope is so cruel that it is incumbent upon us to avoid giving it to others. While it hurts to be rejected in the beginning of an endeavor or relationship, this is nothing compared to the pain of a later rejection. The latter affects our whole person, leading us to doubt and even have contempt for ourselves and others. No one wants to deliver unpleasant news to someone, such as our desire to cut off or not pursue a relationship, but we do more harm by deceiving. The truth often hurts, but we can find ways to make it tolerable.

In what endeavors or relationships have I experienced false hope? How did it affect me?

What do I need to do to recover further? Perhaps I can pray about and dialogue with biblical characters such as Sarah and the wealthy Gentile woman and bring my need for healing and growth to God.

Do I sense any patterns in which I make myself vulnerable to false hope? For example, continually choosing the wrong kind of friends or relationship partners. Do I recognize any self-defeating behaviors or attitudes? How might I alter these?

Am I sensitive to not exposing others to false hope? Am I careful not to mislead others by ingratiating statements that appease rather than candidly communicate or constructively confront?

When I subject others to false hope, do I acknowledge my mistake and try to make reparation?

Saying Goodbye

The Bible is filled with characters who go from one crisis to another. Moses, David, Elijah, Jeremiah, Job, Jesus, and Paul come immediately to mind. The couple who ministered to Elisha's needs experienced the fulfillment of their hopes and the prophecy with the birth of their son, only to have him die suddenly as a child. Here again we have the divine pattern of blessing followed by apparent revocation. The reaction of his mother yields precious insights into the advocacy of motherhood and the credence given it by God.

The Bible describes the death of the Gentile woman's son in a manner that many parents can relate to. Out of nowhere, the child complains of a headache, and before you know it, he is dead. The Bible reports that the mother held the child on her lap until he died at noon.

How many mothers have cradled their dying or still born child in a similar manner. How many children have held their parents in their arms as they died. How many spouses or fiancées have held their partner in their final moments. How many husbands have held their wives after they experienced a miscarriage. How many husbands have opened their arms to their grieving wives on learning that the long hoped-for pregnancy, seemingly indicated by biological signs, was not to be. How many wives have embraced their husband after an employment or business setback. How many parents have hugged their children despite failing marks in school. How many parents have embraced their adult children when their marriage fell on hard times.

The Bible presents a compelling image capable of being transposed onto our lives in many different permutations. Such events occur countless times in human history, and the biblical depiction stands as a universal symbol embracing all other occurrences and inviting prayer, reflection, personal application, and consolation.

One of the most beautiful moments in life is being present to a loved one at death. Particularly therapeutic is the experience of sharing the moment with your mother. She brought you into this world, and now you are privileged to be with her as she leaves it.

Once again, we should not approach this passage with a rigidly literal mind set. There are many persons who have not had the opportunity to cradle or be with their loved one(s) at the moment of death, and they carry this wound for the rest of their life. Such persons can use their faith and imagination and recognize that God and the deceased know of their unfulfilled desire. They can recall all the times they were able to be there for their loved one, when they were even more conscious of it than while drawing their final breaths. They can pray or write a letter sharing their feelings and sit silently while awaiting God's consoling response.

Many emotions come into play during the death of a loved one, usually including a sense of closure and unity. If you have been given the grace to share a loved one's dying moments, you have been blessed by God in a special way.

Have I had the grace to share a pivotal moment with a loved one, particularly but not limited to death? What was the experience like, and how did it affect me?

If I have not been privileged to say goodbye in person to a loved one, I might pray, journal, or write a letter to them and/or God, expressing my sorrow and regrets.

The Father's Respect for Motherhood

When the child first complained of the headache, the first thing the father did was instruct the servant to bring the boy to his mother. I think we can immediately dismiss any notions of a remote, dispassionate father, and instead admire his concern for his wife. Most likely, his thoughts were immediately with her as well as with the boy.

The Bible doesn't tell us whether the father was with the mother as she caressed him in his dying moments, but I think that is a pretty good assumption. What a painful experience that must have been for the both of them. However, at least they could share the pain, whereas Abraham had to deal with the sacrifice of Isaac by himself.

While the Bible focuses our attention on the mother, and our thoughts naturally reside there as well, I think it profitable to consider the grief of the father. After all, he was losing the heir he always wanted, a son to carry on the family name and memory.

I believe there is a level of grief felt by men which goes so deep as to become almost inexpressible. I have undergone experiences that have been so painful that it hurt physically to think about it, and to speak of it would have been unbearable.

Men often seem less capable of coping with deep grief than women. For example, when Job and his wife lost all their possessions and children, Job's wife was immediately able to articulate her grief in succinct fashion, while Job initially sat stoically and presented the image of piety. Only at his wife's prodding was he able to unload his emotions.

How have I coped with my deepest experiences of grief? Have I been able to articulate it verbally and share it with others, or have I found it more bearable to bring it to God in prayer?

Have I tried writing my feelings in a journal? Might I share my entries with a loved one or confidant?

When I have gotten my grief out of my system, was I able to gain some perspective on it?

Not So Fast, God

A mother does not take losing her child easily. Many parents, but particularly mothers, are unable to bear up under the premature loss of their child. We live in a world where children die in ways foreign to the biblical peoples, such as through accidental exposure to poisonous or dangerous materials, kidnapping, reactions to legal and illegal drugs, and fire-arms. This leads us to consider whether the Bible is really relevant to such matters. The reaction of Elisha's Gentile benefactor gives us a conclusive answer.

Any time or way a child dies is indescribably painful to a parent. The Gentile woman exemplifies the spirit of Sarah and mothers throughout history in conveying to Elisha and God that this death is unacceptable.

The Bible's description of this woman leads us to conceive of her as a dynamic, proactive, and persuasive person. Even Elisha could not sustain a no to her, first to her offer of hospitality and then to her request for the reviving of her son. When her child dies she does not hesitate in embarking on the course which seems proper, giving orders to her husband to send for the servant and the donkeys. She is a determined woman of action.

To make a long story short (cf. 2 Kgs 4:8-37), I'll go straight to the story line. After persistent urgings from her for his intercession, Elisha comes to the boy and revives him. Four related points are particularly worthy of our consideration.

It is All Right

First, a frequent theme of this story is that everything is all right. This is what we want to be reassured of during difficult times. Three times in one verse this phrase is used to convey Elisha's concern for the couple and the child (cf. 2 Kgs 4:26).

First, the woman says to both her husband and Elisha that everything is all right. It is as if she expects Elisha and God to hear her prayers. This woman who was so guarded against false hope now acts to mitigate any possibility that she will have hoped in vain. Her determination sheds light on why Sarah was kept in the dark about God's command that Abraham sacrifice Isaac. As discussed in chapter three, she likely would not have stood for it.

God made mothers this way, and He seems quite capable of working with their maternal instincts. A Jewish proverb asserts that God could not be everywhere, so He made mothers.

Second, Elisha observes that God has hidden the boy's death from him, almost as if it is part of the divine plan. We see a similar development in the story of the raising of Lazarus, where Jesus delays in going to see his sick friend, only to receive news that he has died. Jesus proclaims that Lazarus' death is not to be the final word, and that it will witness to the power bestowed on Jesus (cf. Jn 11:14).

Such puzzling events bear reflection. Why does God often operate in such an obscure and protracted manner? We don't have a definitive answer, but the Bible offers clues along with guidance on how God wishes us to cope.

God's mysterious ways of dealing with suffering often evoke turmoil that from our perspective could have been avoided. Clearly, His ways are not ours (cf. Isa 55:8-9). When we don't understand God's seeming silence or inactivity, we need to reach out to each other for help and consolation. That's one reason God gave us each other. He much prefers to work through us, His earthen vessels (cf. 2 Cor 4:7).

Jesus conferred much more power and authority on the apostles than their behavior and capacities would seem to merit. Just as God bragged about Job prior to testing him (cf. Job 1:8; 2:3), God likewise believes in us more than we do, and knows that we are capable of much more than we realize.

Thus the Bible is the potential fulfillment book par excellence. Its primary author gave us our gifts and wants us to realize them fully. He dispenses guidance and encouragement throughout the Bible, and promises to accompany and support us as we try to live it.

God's desire for human beings to come to Him freely, using their gifts creatively and responsibly, permeates the Bible. While He tests us in order to make us better (cf. 1 Pt 1:6-7), we are not to test Him in the sense of abdicating our responsibilities and presuming upon Him to do what we can do. Jesus was tempted to engage in such irresponsibility by throwing himself down from the pinnacle of the temple (cf. Lk 4:9-12).

One of the primary challenges in our potential fulfillment journey is to distinguish between our responsibilities and dependence on providence, as articulated in the Serenity Prayer. The difficulty of maintaining this balance is captured in the spiritual maxim "Act as if everything depends on you, pray as if everything depends on God."

Third, the child is revived gradually, recalling the story of how Jesus healed the blind man through two separate actions (cf. Mk 8:22-26). God often takes His time in healing us. We want instant relief, but God has other plans.

Fourth, Elisha restores the boy to his mother with the words "Take your son" (cf. 2 Kgs 4:36). This succinct exhortation restores the bond and acknowledges the mother's close identification with her son. When Jesus healed a child, he likewise immediately restored the child to its parents (cf. Mk 5:43; Lk 7:15). The dying Jesus told his mother Mary to accept the beloved disciple as her son (cf. Jn 19:26).

All of these points remind us that even in the most tragic of circumstances God has a plan for our welfare. It may include great suffering and even feelings of hopelessness and abandonment on our part. However, we have to believe that God is even more concerned than we are for our well-being, and in His own way and time He will bring it about.

Do I believe that God will make things all right in His time? What experiences have shaped my belief?

Do I believe that God has a plan for my life, including even my daily activities? Do I try to cooperate with this plan through prayer, reflection on the Bible, dialogue with others, and sincere and prudent actions?

What experiences have I had of God taking His time in healing me or loved ones? What happens when I am patient and trusting? How does this facilitate my and others' growth and healing?

Do I identify with my loved ones the way the Gentile mother did with her son? Do I extend my appreciation to loved ones for the way they identify and empathize with me?

When Things Aren't All Right

Not all stories end happily. Things aren't always all right, at least from our perspective. During such times we have to wrestle with this passage and ask God how it applies to our contradictory circumstances. The details and characters change, but the fundamental themes of God's sovereignty and compassion and His receptivity to our persistent pleading remain the same. The woman's dogged determination to accompany Elisha until he gets to the boy brings to mind the righteous persistence of the widow before the corrupt judge in one of Jesus' parables (cf. Lk 18:1-9).

When things aren't all right, do I pretend that they are?

When things aren't all right, do I let God and loved ones know of my anguish?

When things aren't all right for others, do I try to make them right, or at least be there for them?

Each of the biblical stories we have reflected upon has a protracted happy ending. After a lengthy wait and the requisite suspense, God comes through. In the next chapter, we will consider the saga of Jacob, Leah, and Rachel, a story with numerous twists and turns. It ends with sorrow as well as hope. In order to get a balanced perspective on infertility in the Bible and life, we must learn to take the bad with the good (cf. Job 2:10).

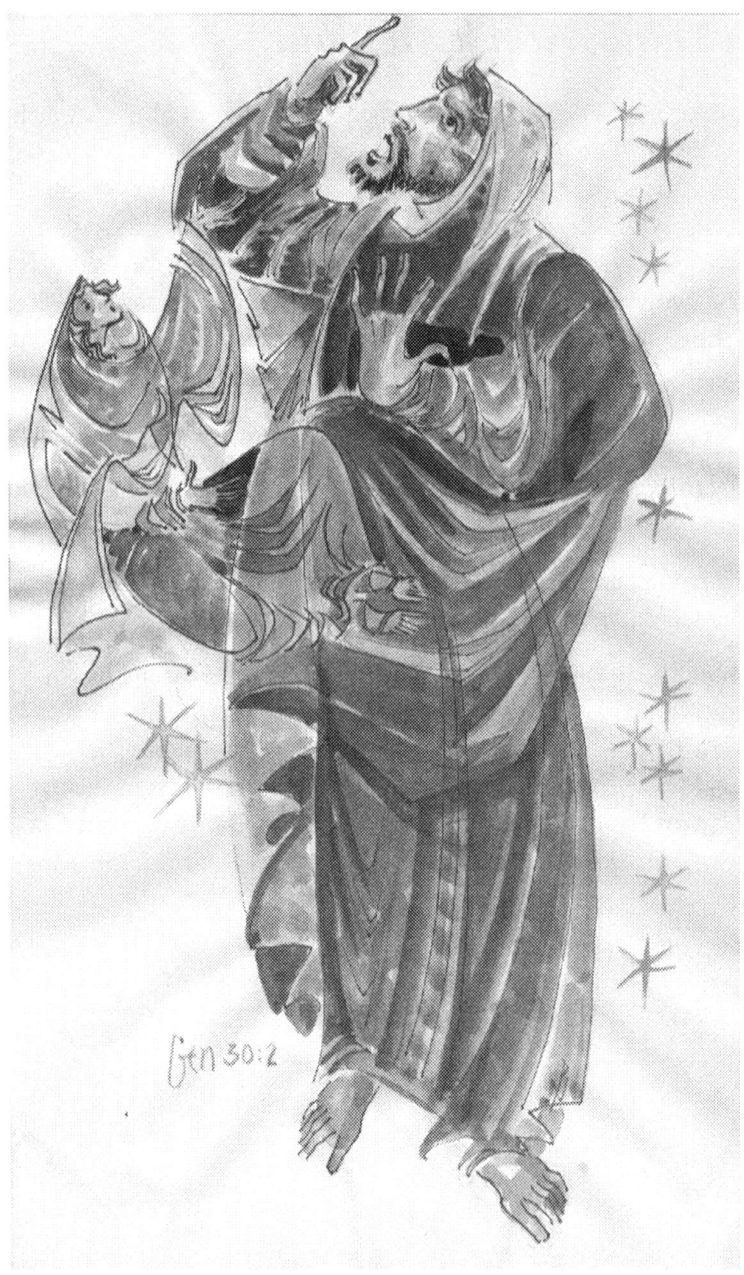

Figure 6. Jacob and Rachel.

The heated conflicts of Jacob and Rachel are a reminder of how infertility can intensify an intimate relationship. Rachel demands children from Jacob, and he asks her incredulously if such is within his power. How easy it is for a wife to expect the impossible from her husband and a husband to lose touch with his wife's feelings and dignity. And vice-versa. The twelve stars signify Jacob's twelve sons, the twelve tribes of Israel, and remind us that God can accomplish His plan even amid human foibles.

Chapter Five

Infertility as a Source of Conflict

Without question the most conflictual experience of infertility in the Bible is that between Jacob and Rachel. It is exacerbated by competition between sisters Rachel and Leah, who double as Jacob's wives. Their quest for offspring, whether through themselves or their maidservant, gives Jacob twelve children, whose lineage would turn out to be the twelve tribes of Israel. The trio's exploits yield profound insight into the human weaknesses that surface during the painful experience of infertility. This is also an example of biblical irony, as Jacob was well-acquainted with sibling rivalry through his struggles with his brother Esau.

Let's set the stage by reviewing Jacob's life and his path to Rachel and Leah.

As we saw in chapter four, Jacob came into this world in a turbulent manner. He struggled with his twin brother Esau as they emerged from their mother's womb, and their rivalry continued throughout adolescence and young adulthood. Nothing unusual there. Their father, Isaac, preferred Esau, while Jacob was his mother Rebekah's favorite.

Jacob exploited Esau's hunger and rash irresponsibility to get his birthright, and at his mother's urging deceived his father and brother and received the paternal blessing normally reserved for the eldest son. This ignited Esau's rage and resulted in Jacob being sent away to his uncle's until his brother's anger subsided. Time and distance was the preferred anger management strategy in those days.

En route, Jacob had a dream in which angels descended and ascended a ladder to heaven, and he was given a promise of God's protection. On his return home he would have another divine encounter, this time in the form of a wrestling match with an angel in which he would prevail. The symbolic import of both have made them among the most famous passages in the Hebrew Bible, and they have direct relevance to all persons on a journey.

In the Bible, God often speaks to men in their dreams. On the symbolic or metaphorical level of interpretation, this may be understood as an appeal to the deepest part of men, the unconscious. Recall that Adam was put into a deep sleep during the creation of Eve (cf. Gen 2:21).

Conversely, with the exception of the wife of Pilate (cf. Mt 27:19), most women are conscious when they are addressed by God, as for example when Mary received the announcement of Jesus' birth from the angel Gabriel (cf. Lk 1:26-38).

Claiming the Divine Initiative

In chapter one, we discussed the foundational spiritual concept, the divine initiative. It is integrally tied to biological and functional fertility, as the ability to produce children and develop ourselves and the earth is bestowed on God's initiative in the beginning of creation. Jacob's two encounters with God symbolize the divine initiative in his and our life. In the first encounter he received God's protection and in the second His blessing. This parallels Jacob's experience with his parents. He was protected by his mother and received a blessing from his father. Our experience of our parents influences our experience of God.

God's protection and blessings bracket the trio's (Jacob, Rachel, and Leah) infertility struggles, which we shall discuss shortly. From a theological and philosophical perspective they frame the context in which our struggles occur, whether they are with biological or functional infertility.

Taking our cue from Jacob's experience, we can infer that God's protection does not insulate us from difficulties, and that His blessings are often accompanied by trials/challenges. The beloved twenty-third psalm captures this: "Even though I walk through the darkest valley, I fear no evil; for you are with me..." (Ps 23:4).

God's blessings and protection is certainly not foremost in most people's mind amid life's obstacles and deprivations. It can be very difficult to believe in God's protection and blessings when circumstances seem to indicate the opposite: that God has abandoned and even cursed us.

This experience is mirrored in the problems germane to marriage—marriage being the primary biblical image of God's relationship with His people. There are times when we feel even those closest to us are not with us, and we are capable of hurting those we love in the deepest way imaginable. The closer we are to someone, whether human or divine, the more vulnerable we become, and the more likely our dark side will surface.

Do I believe that God will protect and bless me amid my experience of biological or functional infertility? In my experience, has He, and if so, how?

In what ways has God not seemed to protect and bless me amid my struggles?

Am I willing to dialogue and wrestle with God when He has let me down and I feel negatively towards Him?

What happens when I bring my anger and doubts to God? (The alternative is to repress or ignore them, and thereby either damage our relationship with God or redirect the negativity towards ourselves or others, who are less capable of handling it.)

Am I willing to forgive loved ones who have hurt me deeply, recognizing that with love comes pain as well as joy?

Am I willing to forgive myself for the hurts I have inflicted on loved ones, both living and dead?

Approaching Infertility in Balanced Fashion

One of the Bible's most consistent as well as maddening attributes is its balance. It presents life in a certain way in one passage or book, then reveals what seems like an opposite perspective in another. It does this because it is true to life and is unafraid to acknowledge and explore life's paradoxical aspects. This reflects its faith in God and confidence in humanity when it cooperates with God.

We see this balance manifested in the ups and downs experienced by biblical characters. For example, Jacob undergoes both inspiring and discouraging experiences. In the process, he grows up and becomes a more spiritual person.

Recognizing the various dimensions of life and the human personality should make us averse to labeling or condemning ourselves or others. Each of us has a good and bad side, strengths and weaknesses. It is misleading and potentially destructive to focus on one to the exclusion of the other.

One of the key benefits of reflecting upon the Bible's infertility stories is that we gain a balanced perspective. We recognize that things are not always black and white, and gradually learn to give ourselves and others the benefit of the doubt and a reasonable amount of leeway. We become measured in our evaluations of situations and persons, and try to look at all sides. We balance principle with practical, personal, and pastoral considerations. In the end, we become more prudent and compassionate, and thus more capable of fulfilling our biological and functional fertility capabilities in a healthy manner.

How might I view my current situation in a more balanced manner? What other perspectives and frames of references could I consider in order to get a more complete picture?

How might I view my weaknesses and shadow side in a positive light? How do they mirror my strengths and offer opportunities for humility, compassion, and growth?

How might I put my strengths in perspective and avoid conceit by recognizing the gifts and support I have received from God and others, particularly loved ones?

Jacob Meets Rachel

The description of the initial encounter between Jacob and Rachel is one of the most romantic in the Bible. After exercising standard ancient near eastern good manners and watering the flock of Rachel's father, as Moses did when meeting his wife Zipporah, Jacob kisses Rachel and weeps for joy.

This passage reminds us how far removed we are culturally from biblical times. Try Jacob's stunt today and you'll get into a different book—down at the precinct for sexual harassment and trespassing.

This passage is important in our struggle with biological or functional infertility because it reminds us of our positive beginnings. It is important that we have a balanced understanding of our closest relationships, including from the perspective of time, and not exaggerate our present problems.

It is important to periodically and particularly during difficult times consider the joy we experienced in our first encounter with our partner or the beginning stages of our personal or professional growth endeavor. This will put our immediate situation in context and perspective and revive positive energies that we can utilize in the present. Otherwise we can become so mired in our negative realities that we lose sight of the positive, which includes the past and future as well as the present.

Alice and Winston

Alice and Winston are upset over their infertility and financial difficulties. They didn't anticipate or talk about these issues prior to their marriage, and now they have to address them under pressure.

Alice and Winston are getting along okay, but their enthusiasm and passion is waning. They need to rekindle the positive feelings that brought them together and stop obsessing over their problems. They can't deny or run away from their plight, but neither should they let it cloud their whole lives and history together.

Alice and Winston established a policy of weekly dates, just like when they were dating. Since they don't have children, this is feasible. Couples with children might have to come up with an alternative arrangement that nonetheless enables them to rekindle their romance.

Alice and Winston occasionally returned to places and activities that carried positive memories, while also seeking out new adventures and locales. It reminded them that they were a gift to each other, and reinforced their positive feelings. This served as a counteractive to the negative feelings that came more from their difficult situation than from any animosity towards each other, and kept these negative feelings from acquiring disproportionate influence.

Bolstered by their renewed appreciation for each other and the identification of the external roots of their discontent, they began making gradual inroads on their difficulties, primarily by conducting an ongoing dialogue that their dates initiated.

How might the image of Jacob joyfully kissing Rachel influence me to rekindle my fondness for my loved one(s)? What can I do to build on the positive memories and put my current difficulties in perspective?

What might be keeping me from returning to positive relationship roots? If I am resistant, why?

The Power of Infatuation

When Jacob encountered his uncle Laban, the two began a discussion about the wages for Jacob's service. Jacob asked for Laban's youngest daughter, Rachel, in exchange for seven years of labor. The Bible reports that Jacob's attraction to Rachel was so powerful that the seven years seemed like only a few days.

This is a classic description of infatuation. This is how we begin relationships, but eventually it wears off. Infatuation rarely endures in the face of infertility, financial and work problems, health difficulties, and in-law problems.

Infatuation is simply the beginning stage of love. It needs to be developed, deepened, and purified, usually through challenging experiences. It is a significant enough experience that in the person of Jacob God ordained that it be pivotal in the development of the Jewish people.

It is important that we recognize that even relationships that start off with a powerful chemistry will eventually encounter disillusionment. Even

God's involvement in the meeting and uniting of two persons doesn't make them immune to eventual or even immediate difficulties.

What is my experience of the power of infatuation?

Do I keep infatuation in perspective and recognize it for what it is, rather than confuse it with love or undersell its natural and necessary preparatory function?

If I feel an attraction in the wrong direction, am I willing to get beyond the initial sensation and recognize its inappropriateness and the consequences of an imprudent response?

In-Law Problems

After Jacob fulfilled his years of service, Laban beat Jacob at his own game and gave him Leah, Rachel's older sister, instead of Rachel. The deceiver got deceived.

Laban is a detestable character who plays with the lives of his kin in order to advance his own interests. He feigns innocence and rationalizes his deception in a way that must have seemed all too familiar to Jacob. Knowing that in an elder-oriented society and in a foreign land he doesn't have much leverage, and wanting Rachel very badly, Jacob agrees to accept Leah and work another seven years for Rachel. Usually it is after marrying his sweetheart that a man becomes a slave to his job, but Jacob had to start early. Jacob's perseverance epitomizes the depth of a man's love for a woman.

Laban's cunning reminds us that in-laws have been making life difficult for couples since time immemorial. In-law relations aren't always troublesome, but they certainly require adjustments on both sides. This isn't the first time in the Bible that shady relatives complicate things for a married couple. Abraham's nephew Lot acted in a dishonorable way towards his uncle by choosing the more desirable land for himself (cf. Gen 13:8-12). In that culture, the younger was expected to defer to the elder.

The tension between Laban and Jacob worsens when Jacob takes off unannounced and unbeknownst to Jacob Rachel steals Laban's household goods. Laban's relatives get involved in the pursuit of Jacob, and a confrontation occurs. Fortunately, God intervened and warned Laban not to say anything to Jacob (cf. Gen 31:24). However the two talked, and hostilities ceased. In-law difficulties get worse as more people and issues become involved. As in Jacob's case, dialogue and distance are usually the appropriate remedy.

Once again it is important to develop a balanced picture of the conflict that develops between Jacob and Laban. Jacob is crafty and knows how to play a situation to his advantage, though with respect to Laban his actions seem mostly honorable.

Laban has his good qualities as well. He eventually gives Rachel to Jacob as promised and makes up with him, but not until he has cheated him several times and only after God has warned him not to harm Jacob. In the end, Jacob and Laban enter into a covenant, an uneasy truce, and each goes their own way. Sometimes that is the best you can do with your in-laws.

Jacob offers a helpful and realistic example for dealing with in-laws. He is patient and respectful, but eventually stands up for himself. He does not hold a grudge, and tries to do what is just. He does not hide behind his wife, as his grandfather Abraham occasionally did (see chapter three). Jacob naturally wants to go back to his own family, but he fulfills his obligations to Laban and his daughters.

The Bible illustrates that of its very nature the in-law relationship can be challenging as well as supportive. In-law problems become particularly thorny when biological and functional infertility issues are involved. Veiled references about the need for grandchildren or financial security come, along with comparisons with siblings who have been gifted with children and / or prosperity. The son- or daughter-in-law becomes not good enough, and tensions mount. Parents don't want to see their children suffer, and when couples undergo difficulties it is natural for parents to be provincial in their sentiments.

Rarely do persons who interfere in or damage a marriage face proportionate consequences. In-laws justify overstepping their bounds and interfering in their offspring's relationship by projecting negativity onto their son- or daughter-in-law. Inevitably one or both partners and any children involved suffer and are left to pick up the pieces.

In-law Implications

Jacob's difficulties with Laban illustrate several common sense principles for dealing with in-laws. First, since like Jacob you don't have your act completely together, you can't expect them to. Tolerance and patience is necessary. Second, when in-laws play too large a role in the lives of their children, distancing needs to occur, even at the expense of hurt feelings. This requires the cooperation of both partners.

Third, respect of in-laws is necessary for maintaining marital harmony. The Bible makes no mention of Rachel's or Leah's resentment of Jacob's attitude and actions, leaving us to infer that in their eyes he acquitted himself well. In stealing her father's goods, Rachel shows she has some of the wiliness of her husband, and that she has sided with him rather than with her father.

It is usually less difficult for a man to create distance from his parents than for a daughter. Parents tend to be more protective of a daughter. We know the old lyric, a son is a son till he takes on a wife, a daughter is a daughter all of her life.

So many common and crucial in-law issues are raised in the saga of Jacob, Leah, and Rachel (cf. Gen 29-31) that we would do well to reflect on it closely. The following questions can help us apply Jacob's lessons to our life.

Do I give my in-laws or my own family the benefit of the doubt and try to approach them with an open, caring mind?

Am I willing to set reasonable boundaries and when chronic transgressions occur uphold them?

In what ways have I put my own interests over others', including my loved ones?

When others offend me, am I willing to consider that my actions may be similar? We reject in others what we dislike in ourselves.

Am I willing to let bygones be bygones and enter into an amicable relationship with in-laws or other family members with whom I have quarreled?

How might I improve my relationship with my partner, in-laws, or family members?

The Unloved Partner

"So Jacob went in to Rachel also, and he loved Rachel more than Leah" (Gen 29:30).

Jacob's first wife, Leah, is a tragic figure who elicits our sympathy. She is used as a pawn by her father in order to get seven years of work out of Jacob, and to her humiliation as the eldest daughter is clearly second to Rachel in Jacob's eyes. The Bible is both subtle and specific in alerting us to the rejection experienced by Leah and her persistent attempts to be loved. Each time she or her maidservant has a child by Jacob she hopes that she will gain favor with him.

There are many Leah's in our midst. Many persons do not feel loved by their partner, and in many cases the partner confirms this by breaking up with or divorcing them. The wound of not feeling loved runs deep, and nothing can take it away. Even moving on to another love does not erase the memory. The unloved person experiences this rejection at the core of their being, and feels incomplete and violated because they are not fully accepted by someone they care deeply for.

Each of us can relate to Leah in some way. We all feel unloved in some relationship or aspect of our personality. Each of us has a void that only God can feel. It is important that we seek fulfillment and healing of this void from God rather than resort to destructive compensating behaviors, chasing after whatever or whoever will mollify our pain.

We also make Leahs out of our loved ones. We reject them outright or leave them feeling not fully accepted. Even when like Leah they do their best to win our affections and approval, it still isn't enough.

Biological or functional infertility can lead to us or our loved one feeling like Leah. It is natural for persons to enter marriage with expectations of children and reasonable financial success, but the lack of either is not sufficient reason to withdraw love from a partner.

Modern Leahs: Ruth and Rolf

Ruth and Rolf seemed to others and themselves a happily married couple. They had their conflicts, but for the most part they were of one heart and mind.

The first few years of their marriage went relatively well. Their care and admiration for each other was obvious, and they enjoyed doing things together. Then, the afflictions came. First, there were health problems. Then came work difficulties and unemployment. Then Rolf began to resent Ruth because she was unable to have a child, even though he knew since they were dating that her cycle was irregular and that she might need medical help to get pregnant.

Rolf began losing patience with Ruth, finding fault with things he had overlooked before. He began to tear down some of the special symbols and patterns they had established together. Ruth took it hard, as she was sentimental and identified intensely with her relationship with Rolf.

The more rejection Ruth felt, the more insecure she became. She began testing Rolf's love, which in turn set off a reaction in him. Soon their conflicts became more heated, and Ruth began withdrawing from the relationship. This infuriated Rolf, who had a fear of abandonment. However, Rolf had triggered this behavior in Ruth by his frequent belittling and distancing, although when he wanted Ruth he expected her to be there for him.

After estrangement set in, they decided to seek counseling. Fortunately, they were referred to a counselor who helped them get out of their cycle of negativity. He guided them in seeking the roots of their problems. Instead of arguing during their session, they discussed things. Instead of recycling grievances, he asked them to recall and count blessings.

The counselor made a point of having them stay positive and build on what brought and held them together. Eventually they would address their immature behaviors and animosities, but for now they were going to learn about themselves. A good therapist can help clients unpack their experiences, emotions, expectations, and grievances, recognize projections and displacements, and distinguish between superficial and essential issues.

The counselor felt that Ruth's infertility was a cause of many of their conflicts. If no babies could be reasonably expected in the near future, they would have to work through it.

The love between spouses should be deepened and expanded by, but not dependent upon, the presence of children. Over-identification with the parental role at the expense of the marital relationship is usually rooted in adolescent experiences and the examples set by parents. As is often observed, one of the best things a parent can do for their children is to love their spouse.

One of the advantages of this discovery-oriented approach is that if the counseling sessions proved unsuccessful, and the couple was unable to overcome their differences, at least they would understand themselves better and not carry as much baggage and projections into their new life apart. One wishes that such separation would not occur, but only the full commitment of both spouses can save a troubled marriage.

Initially Ruth was cast in the role of Leah, but with their fighting and disassociation Rolf likewise began feeling unloved. They are great candidates for reflecting on this passage and identifying with Leah both to heal their own and their partner's wounds.

Reflection on the plight of Leah reminds us that romantic rejection and feeling secondary is a common experience. When we are told that we don't measure up, we should not feel alone. Leah can inspire us to bring our hurt to God, and ask for healing, acceptance, and understanding.

In what relationship or experience can I relate to Leah?

In what relationship or circumstance have I made someone feel like Leah?

Am I willing to direct my need for love to God, rather than rely exclusively on human loves, which are imperfect and fickle?

God Feels Our Pain

> "When the LORD saw that Leah was unloved, he opened her womb; but Rachel was barren" (Gen 29:31).

This one verse of the Bible packs a powerful emotional and spiritual wallop. It contains three main points in tension with each other. First, that God pays attention to our pain. Second, that God will act in His own time. Third, that sometimes our prayers and dreams go unfulfilled, at least for the moment.

It is dangerous to absolutize biblical statements, because each person and circumstance is unique and there are many exceptions to the norm. For example, there are Leahs whose wombs God does not open, whether in terms of not blessing them with children, a suitable partner, or an environment and resources through which they can work towards their potential. There are Rachels—gifted, attractive, and beloved persons—whose womb is not closed, whose efforts at finding a partner, having a child, or fulfilling their potential are not thwarted. Conversely, there are Leahs and Rachels as described in the Bible: women (and men) who are blessed by God amid their forlornness and whose gifts in one area are offset by deficiencies in another area.

What then are we to make of biblical statements and characterizations which may or may not be true in our circumstance?

First, we have to view the Bible as a forum for dialogue with God, others, and ourselves. It is not a book of answers and ready remedies. It is an invitation to persist in our integrity (being ourselves and doing our best) amid our struggles, and to wrestle with God as part of the coping process.

It offers starting points for prayer and deeper contacts with reality. It is a letter from God and our ancestors designed to help us live in a more whole and holy fashion.

The Bible raises questions and offers guidance more than it gives absolute answers, at least in this life, but the process of wrestling with questions leads to responses that can help us in our overall life direction and in our day-to-day living: "So do not worry about tomorrow, for tomorrow will bring worries of its own. Today's trouble is enough for today" (Mt 6:34).

The above succinct biblical observation can help us cope with biological or functional infertility in several ways. First, we can trust that God knows precisely what we are going through and is aware of our real needs: "...for your Father knows what you need before you ask him" (Mt 6:8). A simple but profound prayer like the Lord's Prayer contains all the fundamental spiritual wisdom we need for coping with our difficulties.

Second, we can presume that He will intervene in our lives, even when we are not aware of His actions. This is why discovering and trusting in the divine initiative is such a pivotal step in our spiritual and human development. Such joy comes from those moments when we perceive divine providence at work in our lives!

Third, we need not assume that we are necessarily at fault when doors are closed in our life. Just as Rachel was not responsible for her beauty, Jacob's love for her, and her father's manipulative actions, likewise only God knows why she had to undergo the trial of infertility. However, Rachel's initial infertility reminds us that even the closed doors in our life, be they obstacles to procreation or potential fulfillment, can be stages in God's plan not only to develop and save us and those around us, but in a larger sense, the whole world (cf. Col 1:24).

Do you think Rachel or any of the biblical characters knew of the larger ramifications of their trials at the moment that they underwent them? Did they realize that God was using them to achieve His good purposes? Their reactions indicate that they were like us in focusing narrowly on their own situation, which is natural amid suffering:

> "Now, discipline always seems painful rather than pleasant at the time, but later it yields the peaceful fruit of righteousness to those who have been trained by it" (Heb 12:11).

Remember, the Bible was written much later than the historical events it describes. Its assertions are tinged with hindsight and the fruits of mature reflection and divine inspiration. Likewise God has continued revealing Himself since the composition of the Bible, and we bring greater historical, scientific, and spiritual understanding to our interpretation and application of the Bible. The Bible does not describe static events whose meaning is fixed in history. Rather, it promotes dynamic, unfolding, and personal values which engage individuals and communities in their historical moment and inspire them to open themselves to the love of God and neighbor.

Therefore, a woman unloved by her partner, a man rejected in his profession, parents neglected by their children, a single person unable to find a suitable mate, or anyone in similar circumstances should not consider their situation any less significant in God's eyes and human history than Leah's. Who knows what God has planned for us individually and collectively? Salvation history (God's plan for saving the human race) continues.

A gifted person sidetracked by an unfortunate obstacle or affliction, a person who to others seems to have it all but internally feels deprived of what they want most, a well-meaning person caught up in the machinations of family dysfunctions, can find in Rachel a symbol of their struggle and take their place alongside her in salvation history.

Do these realizations make our sufferings any less painful? Do they make them go away? Do they provide us with assurances that remove our anxieties and fears? Of course not, but they can provide us with the inner peace and consolation of knowing that we are loved and accepted by God even when others, life, or even our own standards and feelings reject us.

We gain this peace beyond understanding (cf. Phil 4:7) by reaching out to the Leahs and Rachels in our midst while asking God and others for help in coping with the experience of Leah and Rachel in ourselves.

In what experiences have I discerned God's noticing of my forlornness? In what circumstances have I felt God's presence when others and life have let me down? How might I draw on this in my present experience of abandonment or rejection?

In what ways has God opened my womb, that is, blessed my biological or functional fertility efforts, particularly when unexpected or during difficult times?

In what ways has God not opened my womb? Have I carried on an ongoing dialogue with Him about this, or have I written Him and/or myself and loved one(s) off and resigned myself to mediocrity?

Am I willing to emulate Rachel in persevering with God and my loved ones even when my gifts in one area are tragically offset by deficiencies in others?

Sibling Rivalry

> "When Rachel saw that she bore Jacob no children, she envied her sister; and she said to Jacob, "Give me children, or I shall die!" Jacob became very angry with Rachel and said, "Am I in the place of God, who has withheld from you the fruit of the womb?" (Gen 30:1-2)

Sibling rivalry has been part of the biblical story from the beginning. It occurred first in Eden, continued during the times of the patriarchs and the Jewish monarchy, and remains with us to this day. Even Jesus was asked to settle a dispute between brothers:

> "Someone in the crowd said to him, "Teacher, tell my brother to divide the family inheritance with me." But he said to him, "Friend, who set me to be a judge or arbitrator over you?" (Lk 12:13-14)

The rivalry between Leah and Rachel is particularly acute because they share a husband and a desire to please him and themselves through children. Rachel has Jacob's affections while Leah has his children. Both want more, and in the end neither will realize their desires completely.

This passage is very helpful for understanding the effect of biological and functional infertility on partners when envy is involved. It is natural for us, particularly for women who are innately socially-conscious, to be aware of how others are faring, especially loved ones. We don't want to fall too far behind or miss out on anything!

Envy results in emotions and negative reactions being misdirected and projected onto innocent parties. Rachel is so upset at being left behind by a sister whom she has gotten used to getting the better of that she wants to die, and in her eyes it's Jacob's fault. Who else can she blame?

At such moments we rarely think clearly and react calmly, whether we are the complainer or the accused. Jacob was also disturbed at not being able to have children with Rachel, but how could he do more than he was doing? Why blame him? Talk to God if you want to vent your frustrations, but don't take them out on me.

The image of Rachel and Jacob at odds over her infertility is one that we can relate to. We can surmise that many of our frustrations with our loved ones, particularly our spouse, originate in issues which are not their fault, but to which they are tied in our eyes.

For example, it is not Rachel's fault that her father is a conniver, but it affects Jacob nonetheless. Who is he going to vent his displeasure towards when Laban is not around? Rachel, of course, because she's the reason Jacob has to deal with Laban. Rachel is going to implicate Jacob in her rivalry with Leah because he's part of the reason Leah has gotten the best of Rachel.

There is just enough logic in these thought processes to enable us to justify our rationalizations and project them onto others, particularly those closest to us—who we typically and presumptively count on to put up with our most eccentric and primitive behaviors. At the core of these projections is an immature, misdirected plea for help and a misguided presumption on our loved one's understanding and patience. Such is better than ignoring or abandoning the person, but a more mature response is possible. The key is to recognize our misguided presumptions and to get our discussion on a calmer plane where emotions can be examined more objectively and tempers and eccentricities kept at bay.

There are countless modern scenarios where the conflict between Rachel and Jacob is re-enacted. A woman is unable to have children at the same time that her siblings are. Her husband has been reluctant to go through all the infertility treatments, and by the time he comes around the woman feels her biological clock winding down. When nothing happens according to her schedule and expectations, who else is there to resent but the man who didn't act proactively or effectively enough?

Naturally he takes her frustrations personally and responds defensively. Soon a blaming, shaming, and framing (projections and displaced emotions) cycle is initiated that incorporates other petty resentments and erupts into a full blown war. All this time neither partner is able to identify the roots of their dissatisfaction as the infertility. Neither wants to admit that they have put their fertility agenda above their marital commitment, rather than as part of it.

Similar frustrations can occur with respect to obstacles to potential fulfillment. For example, the wife gradually comes to realize that her husband is not going to provide for her the way she would like him to, and worse still, in her opinion he's not doing all he can to make things financially better. At first she tries to remember her marital vows and subordinate her financial concerns, but gradually her unexpressed expectations get the better of her and she begins to develop resentment. She also would like him to take a more active role with the children in the areas of discipline, moral and spiritual development, and recreation. Of course, were he to do all these things, he'd have little time and energy left for her and their relationship.

Conversely, the husband finds fault with the wife on many issues: she doesn't prepare meals or maintain the household quite the way he thinks she should. She doesn't attend to the children as he would like. She's put on a few pounds. His chirping at her matches hers at him, and instead of taking quiet time to address their own issues first, they focus on each other's shortcomings as they perceive them.

Neither is intentionally being irresponsible or hyper-critical. Both are operating within such profound constraints and obstacles that they are doing the best they can at the moment, given their immaturities and idiosyncrasies. However, we don't think about this when our expectations are not fulfilled and we find ourselves far behind where we thought we'd be, while our siblings or peers are seemingly doing quite well.

We can imagine ourselves in Jacob's and Rachel's shoes, grieving over their fertility problems and the sibling rivalry that it aroused. We can ask ourselves how they must have felt, and how this relates to our difficulties. What words of advice, consolation, or encouragement might they give us?

We can also give ourselves the benefit of the doubt and be more empathetic about the conflicts that ensue from our biological and functional infertility problems. These difficulties affect us at the core of our being and identity, and it is understandable that our internal and interpersonal conflicts would be intense.

We can take consolation in remembering that Jacob and Rachel and countless others before and after them survived such difficulties and the accompanying scars. "It (love) bears all things, believes all things, hopes all things, endures all things" (1 Cor 13:7). We should never assume that we are deficient as persons or in God's eyes simply because we have difficulty coping with such painful circumstances and at times take our frustrations out on each other.

In what circumstances have I blamed loved ones for issues they have little control over or for which they are sorry?

Are my current frustrations with myself and/or my loved one(s) spurred largely by biological or functional infertility difficulties, over which we have little control? Am I willing to put them in the proper perspective?

Have I secretly blamed and not forgiven myself for whatever role I had in our problems? Would God, or a loved one who truly loves me, want me to continue my self-flagellation?

Determined Mothers

Rachel and Leah are so desperate for children that they resort to having their maids bear them. They follow in the footsteps of their grandmother-in-law Sarah, who likewise displayed the envy shown by Rachel and Leah and sought a practical solution befitting her agenda.

The Bible poignantly illustrates the maternal urge and the determination women show in order to fulfill it. It is an indictment of our materialistic society that so many factors work against motherhood: e.g., stress, greed-driven economic pressures, the increasing social acceptance of divorce, and fathers who are absent due to their own irresponsibility, work pressures, and the injustices of the legal system.

Rachel, Leah, and their servant girls are a poignant symbol of the deep and civilization-enriching drives of motherhood. The twelve tribes of Israel, so crucial in the history of Judaism and western culture, would not have existed were it not for their maternity.

In what ways do I manifest deep drives to fulfill my potential or procreative energies?

Am I supportive of the deep procreative or potential fulfillment urges of my loved one(s)? Is there more that I can do for them?

Unsung Heroes

The Bible rarely says much about the servants of prominent biblical characters, even though they occasionally play a prominent role. This reflects the hierarchical nature of their social structure. However, in God's eyes, the dignity and contributions of those servants is as important as their masters'.

Consider the many persons around us who contribute so much, and are just plain good folks, yet go unappreciated. Consider the anonymity of our own lives, the ignored contributions we make and our talents and efforts that go unappreciated and undeveloped due to the lack of support and opportunities. The Bible is as much about these tragic deprivations as it is about fulfillment. It tells us often that humans judge by appearances, but God sees what humans overlook reads the heart (cf. Mt 6:18; Jn 7:24).

Who are the anonymous persons around me whom I should encourage and support?

What anonymous dimension of my life should I affirm and celebrate, without necessarily calling others' attention to it?

God Achieves His Purposes Amid Our Pain

Eventually Rachel bears a son and names him Joseph. At his birth she cries out that God has removed her reproach, reminding us what a humiliating experience infertility was for an ancient woman, particularly a Jewess. She also immediately prays for another son, thereby affirming how important maternity was to her.

Persons impeded from fulfilling their procreative or developmental potential can identify with Rachel's sense of humiliation and her desire for further vindication. St. Paul referred to an ongoing affliction that he experienced as a thorn in the flesh (cf. 2 Cor 12:7). It has since become a common expression and compelling metaphor in Christian theology for the nagging burdens we experience that God does not remove, but through which He invites our trust:

> "Therefore, to keep me from being too elated, a thorn was given me in the flesh, a messenger of Satan to torment me, to keep me from being too elated. Three times I appealed to the Lord about this, that it would leave me, but he said to me, "My grace is sufficient for you, for power is made perfect in weakness." So, I will boast all the more gladly of my weaknesses, so that the power of Christ may dwell in me. Therefore I am content with weaknesses, insults, hardships, persecutions, and calamities for the sake of Christ; for whenever I am weak, then I am strong" (2 Cor 12:7-10).

What reproaches, humiliations, or thorns in the flesh would I like God to take away?

When God doesn't answer my prayers and mitigate my suffering, how might I cope in a healthy and spiritual manner?

Can I observe any growth or healing that comes from God's ***not*** *removing my affliction, as in St. Paul's case?*

When Last and Least is the Best

Joseph turned out to be the greatest and most influential of the sons of Jacob. In the Bible, the last often finish first in the sense that God works most profoundly through circumstances and persons that seem hopeless.

Joseph was sold into slavery by his envious (seemingly a family trait) brothers and imprisoned in Egypt, but ended up rich and powerful. Like Job (cf. Job 42:7-9), he interceded for those who harmed him. On meeting his brothers after they were delivered into his hands, Joseph uttered one of Scripture's most eloquent and concise observations about divine providence:

> "Do not be afraid! Am I in the place of God? Even though you intended to do harm to me, God intended it for good, in order to preserve a numerous people, as he is doing today" (Gen 50:19-20).

The birth and life of Joseph can inspire us to persevere amid our obstacles in the hope that God will achieve His purposes and bless our efforts, however difficult and unpredictable our journey may be.

Have I had experiences of divine providence in which I survived or prospered amid negative persons or circumstances?

In what circumstances have I felt last and least but through a dramatic reversal of fortunes ended up surprising myself and others? What did I learn from this?

Rachel's Unhappy Ending

In death as in life, Rachel always seemed to come out on top of Leah. The book of Genesis does not tell us about Leah's death, whereas it records briefly but dramatically Rachel's demise. This serves as a fitting conclusion to this chapter, as it dramatizes one of life's inexplicable tragedies: the death of a mother during childbirth.

After so much heartache due to her infertility, Rachel had labor difficulties and died during the birth of her second son, Benjamin. She named him "son of sorrow", but Jacob changed his name to "son of the right", meaning son of his favorite wife, as the right side was considered the preferred or lucky side.

Immediately after her son's birth her midwife encourages her by reminding her that this is another son for her, which she had prayed for after the birth of Joseph (cf. Gen 30:24).

In typical fashion, the Bible describes the death of Rachel succinctly and without extended drama. It leaves it to us to infer the emotions and meaning of such a tragic event. We can use our imagination and recollection of similar circumstances in our life to enter into her and Jacob's experience. Several applications to our reflections on loss and deprivation come to mind.

Lessons of Leah's Life and Rachel's Death

First, death in childbirth was not uncommon prior to the twentieth century. Rachel's death reminds us of the many mothers who died in the act of giving life, and the husbands and children who survived them. What began as a blessed event turned tragic. In one way or another we all have some experience of such turnabouts.

The Bible doesn't tell us if Leah was still living when Rachel died, or of the effects Rachel's death had on Jacob and his children. So great was Rachel's identification with her children that when King Herod slaughtered the infant boys of Bethlehem in hopes of killing the baby Jesus, the New Testament refers to Rachel weeping inconsolably for her children (cf. Mt 2:18; Jer 31:15). The geographical link is that Rachel was buried on the road to Bethlehem.

There is nothing like the death of a mother. As mentioned, one of the greatest graces of life is to be able to be present at the death of your mother. When a mother dies, the family usually splinters, each member going their own way. Mother brought the family together and usually served as the glue that held it together during difficult times. Surviving daughters seem the only ones consistently capable of holding the family together and arranging periodic get-togethers.

Second, and as we have discussed throughout the book, being part of God's plan does not immunize us against pain. We should not interpret tragic or difficult circumstances as de facto signs of God's displeasure or punishment. The story of Adam and Eve reminds us that the tragedy and injustice of life come not from God, but from human disobedience. Fratricide took place within the first family, and ever since violent struggles have been part of human existence, contrary to God's original intentions.

Third, romantic preferences and the rejections that ensue are a natural part of life and do not necessarily have a moral dimension. Jacob preferred Rachel from the time he set eyes on her until his death, and Leah had to live with this. Even the births of her children did not completely compensate for the rejection that she bore. How many persons subsequently have born such rejection, holding onto to the pain in some measure to their grave. Laban was wrong for putting Leah in this situation, but the Bible does not blame Jacob for his preference.

Reflection on Leah's plight can inspire us to persist in life-giving even when our fundamental needs and desires are not met. She symbolizes our unfulfilled hopes and dreams that always remain tantalizingly out of reach. The Bible reports that she had lovely eyes, and with the eyes being the windows to the soul we can infer that she was a tender, sensitive person. The Bible often attributes similar words or actions to them, with the exception being their attitude towards children. While Leah had children partially as a path to her husband's affections, Rachel had them out of her maternal instincts.

Finally, even though we lose a loved one through death or divorce, we need not forget or let go of them completely. We can still preserve their memory in our hearts. Jacob takes care in burying Rachel so that her memory will linger and receive the respect it deserves. Like his wives, Jacob can inspire us by his persistence, as he moves on in God's service even after losing a precious loved one.

What is my experience of motherhood? Do I have wounds that need healing, or memories that bring consolation and inspiration?

With Leah's tragic circumstances in mind, what experiences of rejection and lack of fulfillment might I bring to God for healing? How might recognition of this natural, albeit mysterious and tragic, dimension of rejection enable me to let go of negative feelings about myself and others and move forward?

Am I willing to forgive and accept myself and others when our motives, like Leah's, are imperfect? Only God can judge the heart. What experiences do I need to hand over to God, entrust to His mercy, and stop obsessing over?

Who are the deceased persons in my life whom I most wish to remember? Inspired by Jacob's mourning and remembering of Rachel, what might I say to or about them in prayer, or perhaps in my journal?

With Jacob's persistence and resilience in mind, am I willing to move forward in service of God and my fellow human beings even amid a heavy heart and the recognition that my efforts, though generally well-meaning, are flawed and occasionally destructive? Do I believe that God will bring good out of my efforts and achieve his purposes as He did with the patriarchs and matriarchs?

Despite having two wives and many sons, Jacob had to bear much of his sorrow alone. The biblical characters we will encounter in our next chapter, Hannah and Elkanah, had each other for consolation, though like her matriarchal predecessors, Hannah was able to find little comfort even in the love of her caring husband.

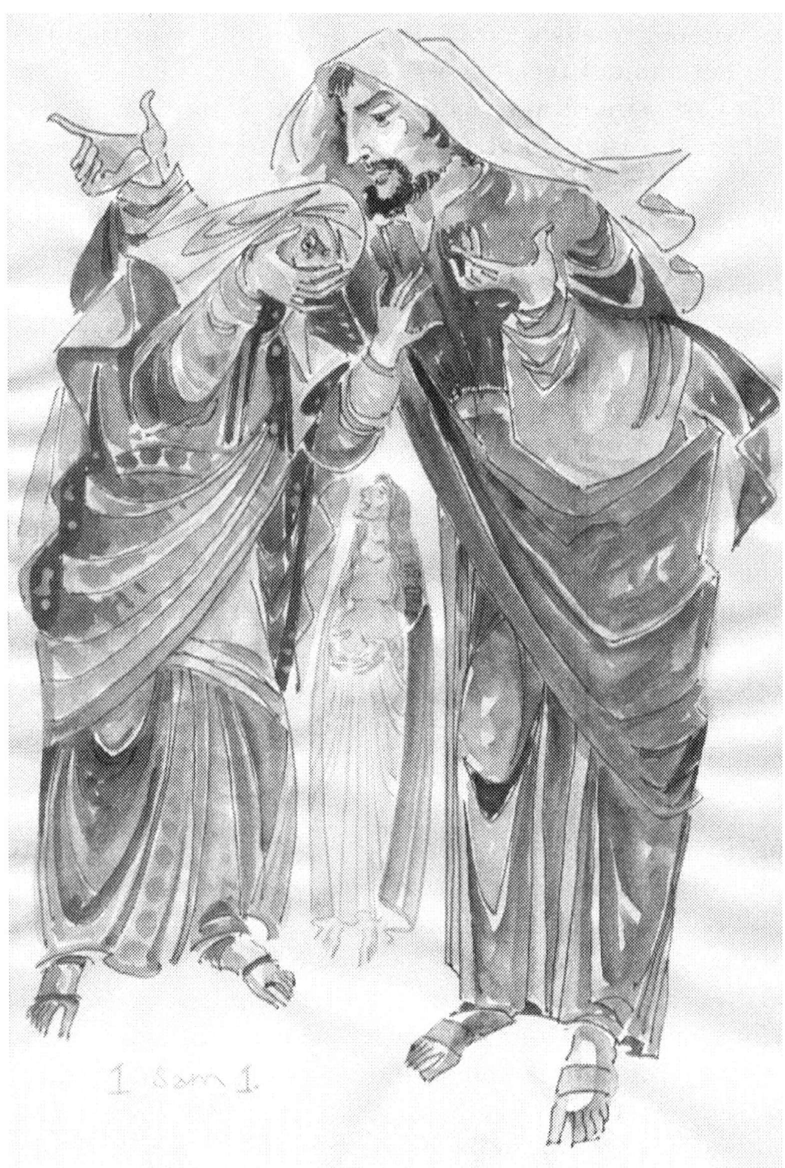

Figure 7. Elkanah, Hannah, and Penninah.

The circumstances surrounding the infertility of the parents of the prophet Samuel recall the past and have a timeless element as well. The last parents recorded in the Old Testament as struggling with infertility, their plight brings to mind the struggles of their predecessors. The rivalry of Sarah and Hagar, and Rachel and Leah pales in comparison to that between Hannah and Peninnah, where resentment and ridicule lead to uncontrollable tears and depression. Peninnah is second in her husband's affections to Hannah, just as Leah was to Rachel and Hagar to Sarah. Peninnah responds inappropriately to her functional infertility by bringing others down with her. Misery loves company. Hannah's grief and marginalization of Elkanah may be excessive, but her turning to the Lord amid her struggles is a model for us.

We know how tempting it is amid either biological or functional infertility to exploit the advantages we gain at the expense of the vulnerabilities of others, and to agitate rather than comfort them. If only we could overcome our insecurities and disappointment and trust that there are redemptive and therapeutic possibilities attached to the thorns we encounter in the most intimate parts of our being and relationships (cf. 2 Cor 12:7-10).

The derisive finger-pointing of Peninnah, born of envy and insecurity, and the abject depression and narrow focus of Hannah illustrate dimensions of the woman's experience and perspective amid infertility. The fruitless attempt of Elkanah to remind Hannah that his presence ought to be worth ten sons exposes male insecurities and insensitivities. Neither gender understands the other, or themselves for that matter. If not for divine and human intervention, infertile couples would have little hope. However, the tenderness, gentleness, and submissiveness of this holy couple remind us that through the practice of perseverance and virtue, infertility in whatever form and circumstance can be endured, and God can bring good out of it in His own way and time. In the Bible, for example at the Sea of Reeds (cf. Exod 15) and at the altar of Moriah where Isaac was to be sacrificed (cf. Gen 22), God often waits until the last minute to deliver his people from harm, so we must be patient.

Chapter Six

The Consuming Sorrow of Infertility: Making Infertility a Shared Experience

Throughout this book we have surveyed both uplifting and sobering aspects of biological and functional infertility. It can unite couples and bring out the best in the human spirit, or it can lead to depression, anger, conflict, and division. In this chapter, we will reflect on perhaps the most touching tale of biological infertility in all of literature. It is an important story within the Old Testament, but is less well known than the stories discussed previously.

1 Sam 1-2 is the story of Elkanah, Hannah, and Penninah, a threesome living in the late eleventh century, B.C. They bring to mind Jacob, Rachel, and Leah: Hannah was infertile while Penninah bore Elkanah children, but Hannah was loved more by Elkanah.

Every year Elkanah would make the trek to the temple to worship and offer sacrifices, and Hannah would receive a better gift to offer because she was his favorite. However, this did little to console Hannah in the face of Penninah's frequent taunts about her infertility.

The story is just beginning and we are already encountering universal human behaviors. Romantic preferences trigger a sense of rejection in Penninah, who in turn evokes feelings of rejection in Hannah by exploiting her infertility.

Rejection

Rejection is one of the most difficult human experiences. Dr. Herbert E. Thomas has written an excellent book entitled *The Shame Response to Rejection* (Albanel Publishers, 1997) in which he details the physical as well as emotional and spiritual effects of rejection. Rejection can evoke an experience of shame that unless understood and addressed properly can result in violence directed towards oneself or others.

How do I typically respond to rejection?

What experiences of rejection triggered a sense of shame (feelings that I don't fit in and am unwanted and unworthy) in me? How might acceptance, albeit reluctant, of the inevitability of rejection in a world of preferences help me to not take it as personally and to gravitate towards persons and environments where I am accepted?

When I feel ashamed, how do I respond? Do I strike out against myself or others? How might I cope more effectively?

Feminine Rivalry

In the last chapter we noted that women tend to be more socially conscious than men and more aware of how they are perceived by others. We need only look at the world of fashion to see the importance placed by women on their appearance and others' opinion of them.

Consider then the damage caused by Penninah in her tormenting of Hannah. The Bible doesn't specify how she went about this, but my intuition is that it was subtle and cutting in a way we would call passive aggressive.

Knowing that Elkanah favored Hannah, Penninah would be wise to not be blatant in her provocations. However, given men's obliviousness to women's indirect messages, she probably could have been obvious and still escaped Elkanah's notice. Hannah's natural feminine sensitivity would likely have been heightened by the insecure feelings accompanying her infertility, and she would not have missed any of Penninah's subtle messages.

Just as each of us tends to be our own worst enemy, so the genders tend to be their own worst enemy. This is particularly true with respect to gender-sensitive issues such as biological and functional infertility.

Except when they are being intentionally hurtful, men rarely make infertile women feel bad about their infertility. When they make an unthinking or insensitive remark the woman usually recognizes that they don't mean anything by it. However, a woman feels that her female peers or family members should know better, and may be trying to make a competitive or personal statement by references to her infertility. Such remarks typically offend and cut deep.

It is usually not our own sex in general that proves to be our rival or tormentor. It is persons close to us who are most capable of inflicting or deepening wounds.

Rarely do we set out to be cruel to loved ones. Rather, insecurities, defensiveness, and competitiveness/ego come into play and influence us to act out of immature and often aggressive self-centeredness rather than compassion and prudence.

Penninah resents being second banana in love, and in that culture she couldn't easily walk away from her marriage. She compensates by projecting her anger and insecurities onto Hannah and making life miserable for her. We can imagine her harshness as a resentful romantic rival with few palatable options and outlets at her disposal. Hannah, being a sensitive woman not inclined to retaliation, takes it to heart. She weeps constantly and will not eat.

I don't think we should be too quick to make Hannah above reproach. She had her faults like the rest of us, and undoubtedly some of these grated on Penninah. However, as often happens in life, the aggrieved person overreacts and exceeds the boundaries of justice and fair fighting.

By recognizing that Hannah is as fragile and imperfect as us, we can identify with her and let her example inspire us to avoid retaliation and instead take refuge in prayer and trust in God. It was probably no easier for her than it would be for us. The suffering she endured is a realistic reminder that a virtuous and spiritual response to injustice and deprivation will not necessarily reduce our pain. Rather, it transforms it into a seed of growth through one's trust in God and acceptance of divine providence.

When Elkanah notices Hannah's grief he experiences a touch of insecurity and rejection as well. Doesn't she have me? Aren't I worth as much to her as ten sons? His reaction lends insight into the typical male response to both biological and functional infertility, as we will now discuss.

In what way am I like Hannah, experiencing torment at the hands of an aggrieved rival? Is my response similar to hers?

In what way am I like Penninah, responding to rejection with envy and bitterness? Who are the Hannah's in my life, and how might I relate to them more compassionately?

In what way am I like Elkanah, wanting to be loved and placed first, yet also having to recognize the other needs and desires of my loved one?

Men's Response to Infertility

Let's first consider the male reaction to biological infertility. It is common knowledge that in their initial stage of grieving men are less demonstrative and passionate in their expressions. The book of Job illustrates this through Job's initial piety in the face of disaster. His wife speaks for women everywhere in criticizing him for his stoicism (cf. Job 2:9).

Elkanah's words and attitude aptly capture the male reaction to infertility and a grieving wife. The first thing a husband thinks about is the reaction of his wife, who is usually crestfallen. He tries to reassure her and doesn't want to see her cry, though that may be just what she needs at the moment.

Usually a man will hug or touch his wife in some way so as to communicate caring. His usual mistake is to stop his physical outreach too soon and instead try to comfort with words that fail to address the depth of the interior wound. A woman needs comforting words, but only after she has sufficiently felt her partner's touch and presence, and has had an opportunity to express her feelings. Then she is ready to listen.

There is nothing like a good, shared cry to help a woman feel she is not alone. This is what Mrs. Job was looking for from Job, not some pious words that don't do justice to the tragedy of the situation.

Infertility creates a sinking, empty feeling in your stomach. You feel cheated and deprived. Why am I denied what comes so easily to others? These feelings intensify if you are trying to lead a good life and feel that fertility should be one of the rewards. Then you begin to build resentment and look for someone to blame. God is a good target for venting your frustrations and anger, but unless you are willing to sit still and listen for His response, usually in the form of a calming presence and discernible intuitive directives or reminders, you are likely to experience it as little more than a release.

Part of the male reaction to infertility comes from socialization. Men are conditioned to appear strong and in control. Some men view demonstrative grieving as a sign of weakness and femininity. In fact, others often need them to be strong and stable, so that they can cope with their own grief. However, men still need an outlet and forum for their grieving.

Unfortunately, men's desire to be there for others or simply to look composed can lead to repression and misdirection of emotions and the conveyance of an emotional coldness that alienates women, particularly their partner.

A man's initial inclination in response to infertility, like most problems, is to think or act (i.e., muster a practical response) his way through it, while a woman feels and talks her way. Accordingly, they are prone to misunderstand each other. The man feels insecure about the woman's failure to acknowledge his importance to her, while the woman thinks the husband is insensitive to her feelings and perhaps doesn't care that much about having the child.

A husband wants to be first in his wife's eyes. It is hard for him to understand the deep drive to motherhood, which at times seem to obscure her vocation as a wife. Reflecting this, Elkanah asks why he isn't enough. He speaks for husbands everywhere in posing the classic question: "Am I not more to you than ten sons?" (1 Sam 1:8). Hannah doesn't answer because there is no answer. The emptiness and pain is that deep. The only suitable response to such anguish is compassionate presence, literally being with someone in their pain.

Integrating the Human and Divine Planes

> "After they had eaten and drunk at Shiloh, Hannah rose and presented herself before the LORD" (1 SAM 1:9).

Apparently Elkanah succeeded in getting Hannah to eat and drink. This is not an incidental detail, as God usually heals in the Bible through the natural world. For example, after reviving a little girl who had died, Jesus instructs her parents to give her something to eat (cf. Mk 5:43). When healing a blind man, Jesus uses saliva (cf. Mk 8:23).

Sometimes spiritually-inclined people move too swiftly to the spiritual realm when attempting to help someone. The natural world is intimately tied to the spiritual, and reaching out to someone on the human level can be a profound spiritual act. People will pray and read the Bible better if they have enough food and drink to sustain them in those activities.

In the last judgment parable in the Gospel of Matthew (cf. Mt 25:31-46), Jesus identifies responses to human needs (feeding the hungry, giving drink to the thirsty, clothing the naked, welcoming strangers, visiting the sick and prisoners, etc.) as the criteria for salvation.

In what circumstances have I opted for a spiritual remedy such as prayer or spiritual counsel when my first response should be on the human plane?

When others have spiritualized issues when I needed a more human response, am I willing to understand and forgive?

In what current circumstances are there practical human responses I can make to help or heal others or myself?

How do I feel when I help or am helped on the human plane?

Going to God for Strength

In the Lord's Prayer, Jesus advises his followers to petition God for their daily bread, that is, sustenance for the day. He most likely means this on both a human (temporal needs) and spiritual (an implicit reference to the Eucharist, the bread of life; cf. Jn 6) plane. Hannah integrates both forms of nourishment by following her eating and drinking with presenting herself before God and engaging in deep prayer and mourning.

As people in grief are wont to do, she bargains with God and promises to dedicate her desired son to God.

A priest sees her moving her mouth silently in prayer in the manner of that day and presumes that she was drunk. After being rebuked by the priest, Hannah corrects his perception and responds that she is "pouring out my soul before the LORD" (1 Sam 1:15). What an apt description of an efficacious spiritual response to infertility, whether biological or functional.

We should also note that Hannah was misunderstood and criticized when she was trying to do good. Appearances can be deceiving, and most people react to initial, surface impressions. We should not be surprised when we are misjudged in our efforts to respond properly to our biological or functional infertility challenge.

Hannah manifests the ideal holistic response to loss and deprivation. She addresses her human needs, then turns to God with her whole self. If you have ever tried to mouth or whisper words while you read, you will realize that it requires additional energy and gets your sense of speech, hearing, touch, and taste (in both the metaphorical and physical sense of tasting the words) involved.

Hannah gives her whole self to God, yet initially receives a rebuke in response. However, God can use human misperception as part of His plan.

Hannah's response encourages me because I get tired of praying and receiving no acceptable response. I get worn down by the same daily struggles and seeing my way barred because of unfortunate circumstances that I can do little to change.

Sometimes I muster the strength to pray a relevant Bible passage (e.g., a complaint to God such as found in Job, Jeremiah, or the Psalms), and when I do I usually find consolation or at least a therapeutic release and a deep sense of peace. My problems remain, but my perspective on them broadens, and I find the strength to persevere.

When I am in crisis, do I turn to God with my whole self, or do I over-indulge in temporary relief measures such as television, sexual stimulation, idle conversation, and food?

Am I willing to put more energy into my prayer so that more of myself enters into intimate contact with God? For example, I can whisper or pray aloud, sing, use hand gestures, or kneel. If I am angry and frustrated, I can shake my fist at God, then imaginatively give Him a tension-relieving, bone-crushing hug. Better to take my frustrations out on Him, who can handle them, rather than on myself, a loved one, or an innocent bystander.

Painful Misunderstandings

I can also relate to Hannah being misunderstood by the priest.

Not only in a parallel fashion, but literally. I've had clergy and other spiritual people mistake my motives or express what I felt were unfair presumptions or judgments. In trying to live a spiritual life and interact respectfully with others doing the same, we discover that good intentions do not eliminate human foibles and the hazards of relating closely to others.

I have been rejected and put-down by people who judged based on appearances and their own bias. They were unwilling to take the time to examine my situation and consider my perspective, much less offer practical assistance. Conversely, the more you get your hands dirty and your ears wet in reaching out to others, the less easy answers and rash judgments you are inclined to offer. Human interactions and affairs are inherently messy, and if I am expecting perfection I can also expect disappointment and conflict.

Of course, I've also been on the dispensing end of criticism and counsel, dispensing it to others based on my agenda and projections rather than a real desire to help them in the way they need it. Most of us have been both the overwhelmed sufferer and the remote but critical observer.

As I share some of the ways I feel an affinity with her experience, I have a hunch you'll recognize parallels in your experience as well.

The infertile couple sometimes gets the following counsel from friendly advice-givers: "just have a bottle of wine and relax." That may work on occasion, but usually a more sustained and scientific remedy is necessary. Or else they hear "why not adopt?", their advisor not realizing that such is difficult financially and emotionally for some couples.

Good counselors withhold advice until they know as much of the whole story and various sides as possible. Their counsel is usually measured, and is issued in a dialogical rather than in a coercive, dogmatic, and judgmental manner. Their compassion, sensitivity, and prudence prevents them from issuing facile, simplistic suggestions that offend rather than affirm. In most cases they try to help the person(s) arrive at their own decisions, as they are most familiar with their own circumstances and capacities.

Am I willing to trust in myself, and if applicable, my partner, when I/we run into procreative and potential fulfillment obstacles, while being humbly and prudently open to competent counsel and support?

Am I willing to overlook the imprudence of others and forgive them for providing easy answers to my complex problems?

When have I oversimplified the circumstances of others and issued misguided counsel or criticism? If feasible, am I willing to express my regret to them?

Am I willing to persevere amid criticism, imprudent counsels, insensitive comments, cutting remarks, and discouraging setbacks, confident that God will eventually reward me for my steadfastness: "And without faith it is impossible to please God, for whoever would approach him must believe that he exists and that he rewards those who seek him" (Heb 11:6)?

Deeply Troubled

Hannah tells the priest that she is deeply troubled and is speaking out of anxiety and vexation. Similar words are used to describe the experience of Jesus in Gethsemane. He knew functional infertility in a very real way. His mission resulted in his being rejected by the people he came to save, crucified by the civil authorities at the urging of the religious leaders, abandoned by his closest followers, betrayed by one of his own, and perhaps most painfully of all, being misunderstood by his family, friends, and neighbors. So great was his dismay over their non-receptivity that he had difficulty working miracles among them (cf. Mk 6:4-5).

Jesus also knew biological infertility in the sense of not having the companionship and support of a wife and children, something that was standard fare for Jews of that period.

Many biblical characters responded positively to deeply troubling experiences. David repented of his adultery and composed one of the most moving and influential psalms in the Bible (Psalm 51). Jeremiah almost despaired of God's help yet uttered the most important prophetic passage from a Christian perspective in the Old Testament, Jer 31:31-34. It is the longest Old Testament passage quoted in the New Testament (cf. Heb 8:8-11). Job lashed out at God amid his agony and uttered profound and consoling insights into suffering. Mary and Joseph were troubled by the mysterious, unprecedented nature of Jesus' birth and by the misunderstandings that accompanied their raising of Jesus (cf. Mk 3:21; Lk 2:48-51; Jn 2:1-5).

We should not deem our response to our troubles any less important in God's eyes. The biblical characters referenced above were using their gifts to the best of their ability, and we can do the same. That is all God asks.

When Jesus was looking for someone to praise and hold up as an example he picked such nobodies in that society as children (cf. Lk 18:17), a widow (cf. Lk 21:1-4), a sinful woman (cf. Lk 7:44-50; Mk 14:3-9), and a tax collector, Zacchaeus (cf. Lk 19:1-10). He picked humble fishermen for his followers.

Old Testament heroes likewise had humble beginnings. David tended sheep, the youngest of eight boys. Amos was a shepherd without the customary priestly training expected of prophets in those days. Jacob was a refugee and his son Joseph was sold into slavery by his brothers.

Do I believe that God holds my faithfulness amid difficulties in high regard? Do I believe that He will bestow honor, glory, and peace on me in His own time (cf. Rom 2:6-11), just as He did with the biblical heroes?

Do I point out to others the nobility of their efforts even when society does not regard and affirm them as such?

God Answers Hannah's Prayers

By now you are accustomed to patterns and themes being repeated in the Bible. Sarah and Abraham received word from an intermediary that she would bear a son, and now Hannah receives a similar impromptu prophesy from the priest Eli. Her response will be echoed by Mary on receiving news from the angel Gabriel that she will bear Jesus. Both proclaim themselves a servant of the Lord.

The words Hannah prays when she has her son (cf. 1 Sam 2) were likely the inspiration for what has become known as the Magnificat (from "My soul *magnifies* the Lord"), Mary's prayer in response to the angel's prophesy (cf. Lk 1: 46-55).

Recognizing such continuity in the Bible is the first step in discovering its continuity with our lives individually and collectively.

What words do you have for God when He answers your prayers today, even in small matters?

Renewed Hope

> "Then the woman went to her quarters, ate and drank with her husband, and her countenance was sad no longer" (1 Sam 1:18).

Hannah was so consoled by this unexpected prophesy that she was able to desist from her mourning and put on a happy face. Our face reveals so much of our emotions. What joy underlies these few words in the Bible, words that convey the revived hope of a woman desperate to exercise her maternity.

Do you know individuals similarly anxious to exercise their maternity and paternity? Do you pray for and try to support them?

Do you know persons desperate to exercise their functional potential, whether that means going to school, embarking on a career, working in a meaningful job, or doing volunteer or ministerial work? Do you pray for and try to support them?

If you are one such person, do you pray for hope and open your eyes to signs of God's caring presence? Do you ask for others' support when necessary?

Do you celebrate the rays of hope that God shines forth, even when they are not the rainbow you seek?

Are you willing to pursue your rainbow amid the clouds, and accept God's will when He has a different sort of rainbow in mind for you?

How wonderful it is when God intervenes in our lives, usually through other persons, nature, and unexpected events. God gives hope, something persons impeded from fulfilling their procreative and functional potential desperately need.

How important it is that we give hope to each other through caring words, gestures, and actions. When I give hope to someone, I am like an angel, which means messenger. I become the hands and feet of God.

To whom might I give hope today, even in a small way?

Sharing the Joys and the Pains

After Elkanah initially tried to console Hannah with affirmation of his presence, the Bible says that they ate and drank, without mentioning Hannah by name. Now that her hope is renewed, the Bible specifically mentions Hannah's restored appetite and includes the detail that she ate with her husband.

This succinctly illustrates the importance of sharing our biological and functional struggles with our loved ones. Can you imagine the dried tears on Hannah's face, her radiant smile, and the relaxed nature of her body? Can you see the furrowed brow and exaggerated wrinkles disappear from Elkanah, his perplexed, worried look a thing of the past?

These concise biblical details are meant to spawn our imaginative reflection and personal applications.

Do you remember going for a ride or sitting down for a meal or a drink with someone in celebration, perhaps after taking a test, finishing a project, or getting good results on a medical check-up? When you are down, it is helpful to be reminded that life contains joyful moments along with its sorrows. We need only review our past and present to rediscover this.

Do you remember sharing a meal or moment amid an unhappy situation, when your and their presence meant so much?

Do you believe that God wills happy experiences for our sustenance, and sad experiences so that we will grow in virtue? Which of your experiences confirm or contradict this?

Pay attention to the facial gestures and body language of others, particularly loved ones. We communicate as much with these as with our words. Who needs your celebratory or consoling presence and support today? Whose do you need?

Have you told persons who have been present to you amid your pain how grateful you are?

Happy Endings and Promise Fulfilled

> "Early the next morning they worshiped before the LORD, and then returned to their home in Ramah. When Elkanah had relations with his wife Hannah, the LORD remembered her. She conceived, and at the end of her term bore a son whom she called Samuel, since she had asked the LORD for him" (1 Sam 1:19-20).

Hannah does not cease praising God once her celebration is ended. She is a consistent servant of the Lord, exemplifying the reverent perseverance necessary for enduring the terrible trials of whatever form of infertility we bear. If we continued with the story we would discover that Hannah made good on her end of the bargain, dedicating and raising her son as she promised.

Her son Samuel became a judge (leader) of Israel who anointed Saul and David as kings. He thereby inaugurated the monarchy. Samuel would emulate his mother in being faithful to God's call, and as discussed in chapter 3 he is one of the few biblical characters to have his name repeated during a summons from the Lord (cf. 1 Sam 4). The exclusive company he attained in God's eyes is captured in the following revelation given to Jeremiah:

> "Then the LORD said to me: Though Moses and Samuel stood before me, yet my heart would not turn toward this people. Send them out of my sight, and let them go!" (Jer 15:1)

The point is that God often rewards our fidelity amid suffering with equally profound gifts and joys that benefit others as well. As specified by Paul in Col 1:24 and as discussed in the beginning of the next chapter, our faithful perseverance amid suffering plays a significant role in God's plan for saving the world. This makes our lives meaningful not only with respect to this world, but the next. In the Bible and life, God consistently implements His saving plan and actions through persons and situations society and often we ourselves consider hopeless and cursed.

When have I been an instrument of God's love and mercy despite my feeling disappointed about my situation and behavior? In which of my experiences has God brought silver linings into dark clouds?

Do I look down on persons who are different from me and whom I find displeasing? Do I discount their role in God's saving plan? If so, what is the root of my insecurity and condescending attitude?

As I observe long-suffering biblical characters such as the patriarchs and matriarchs, the anonymous mother of Samson, the rich woman who assisted Elijah, and Hannah and Elkanah finally have their prayers answered by God, and in a most splendid way, I take courage that God will eventually vindicate my efforts and bless me in a way far beyond my imagination. Perhaps it won't happen in this life. Perhaps my blessing will be received mostly by others. Still, I hope amid hopelessness (cf. Rom 4:18), because I never come to the conclusion that my efforts are in vein.

If I am unable to have a child or find a partner, I keep trying and praying.

If I am unable to make a decent living, I try new things and persist in what I am good at.

If I am unable to reconcile a relationship, I try not to retaliate in word or deed.

If I am rejected by a loved one, I put it and them in God's hands and pray for healing.

If by age, illness, or oppression, I am prevented from doing what I could before, I creatively try to thrive as I am.

Do my positive attitude and actions take away my pain? Of course not. Do they erase the sad memories? Of course not.

However, they do put my struggles in perspective such that I am able to focus on what I have and what is within my means and capabilities.

Does this mean that God wants me to have undergone my unbearable burdens for their own sake or out of some thirst for reparation? Of course not. However, I affirm Job's words on coming out of his struggles and his encounter with God (cf. Job 42:1-6), that God is all-powerful and all-knowing, that He is accomplishing His will despite human opposition and through human cooperation, and that by experiencing His presence/grace I have the strength I need to not only survive but thrive in God's eyes.

I am sure that the biblical characters who bore unbearable burdens spent many a moment wondering whether it was all worth it. Jesus captures the poignancy of our experiences of suffering, waiting, and celebration:

> "Very truly, I tell you, you will weep and mourn, but the world will rejoice; you will have pain, but your pain will turn into joy. When a woman is in labor, she has pain, because her hour has come. But when her child is born, she no longer remembers the anguish because of the joy of having brought a human being into the world. So you have pain now; but I will see you again, and your hearts will rejoice, and no one will take your joy from you" (Jn 16:20-22).

Do I believe that God will reward me in the end, and that I will be satisfied? In what experiences have I received a foreshadowing taste or glimpse of God's gracious rewards?

When I have gotten discouraged and responded destructively, am I willing to turn to God and others for help and forgiveness?

Do I have reasonable expectations for myself and others, so that when I or others fall en route I respond compassionately and resiliently?

Do I observe, admire, and reflect upon inspiring persons in my own era and right in my midst, and draw strength and insight from their examples?

Do I draw strength from my own efforts, remembering how I was able to overcome obstacles in the past and trust that God will help me do so again?

Do I recognize that the ultimate obstacle and enemy is the temptation to give up? If I continue to try, then I am on the path to victory, if not in this world's eyes and context, but in God's.

Coping and Hoping Together

Hannah and Elkanah worship together, then return home. These are not insignificant details, particularly in a culture where for a long time women worshiped in a separate part of the temple from their husband. The couple that prays and journeys together most often stays together. Hannah and Elkanah present an inspiring model for working through fertility and potential fulfillment issues in a united manner.

Another biblical couple that share their spirituality is Tobias and Sarah. (The book of Tobit is part of Catholic and Orthodox Bibles, but is placed in the Apocrypha or disputed books by Protestants. Jews do not include Tobit as part of their Bible.) Their wedding night prayer is one of the most inspirational and timeless in the Bible. In today's egalitarian environment, a couple could pray this without flinching:

> "Blessed are you, O God of our ancestors, and blessed is your name in all generations forever. Let the heavens and the whole creation bless you forever.

You made Adam, and for him you made his wife Eve as a helper and support.

From the two of them the human race has sprung.

You said, 'It is not good that the man should be alone; let us make a helper for him like himself.' I now am taking this kinswoman of mine, not because of lust, but with sincerity.

Grant that she and I may find mercy and that we may grow old together."

And they both said, "Amen, Amen." Then they went to sleep for the night" (Tob 8:5-9).

Do I share my spirituality or journey with loved ones? Do I try to go it alone? What happens when I do either?

Do I monitor how my loved ones are doing on their journey, or am I totally engrossed in mine?

Do I make it a point to do essential activities with my loved one(s)?

Presence

In closing this chapter, it is fitting that we ponder the significant detail that the Lord "remembered" Hannah. Remembering in the Bible is an active understanding of dynamic presence. It is participative rather than passive, and present-oriented rather than nostalgic. It is a reliving, and not just a retelling.

In Lk 23:42, the repentant thief on the cross asks Jesus to remember him when Jesus enters his kingdom. When Jews celebrate the Passover, and Christians celebrate the Lord's Supper, they re-enact the meal as if it re-occurs, as if God is present in a special way and they are participants in the original event.

The word religion comes from the Latin *religio*, which means to rejoin. True spirituality unites us with God, our true self, our neighbor, and the rest of creation. The devil, whose name in Greek means to divide or slander, comes to scatter and disengage. Accusations and adversarial actions (the Hebrew meaning of the name Satan) push us apart.

Oh God, remember us when we struggle with infertility of any sort and other losses and deprivations. God, help us to remember others in their struggles.

Teach us to be present to you and to others, so that we may find the strength we need to endure our unbearable burdens.

Do I remember others, particularly loved ones, amid their struggles, making a point to be as present to them as I can?

Do I invite others to be present to me when I am in need?

Will I forgive myself and others for the times we are not present to each other?

As discussed earlier, the story of Mary and Joseph in the New Testament has several similarities to that of Elkanah and Hannah. Both are pious couples who receive prophecy of the birth of a child. Both are misunderstood because of others' superficial, uninformed judgments. (Mary was undoubtedly the subject of gossip for being pregnant before her marriage to Joseph was consummated by her being brought into his home.) Both are parents of a very influential and holy son. Both women express their gratitude to God in moving and articulate fashion.

However, it is the story of Mary's cousin, Elizabeth, and her husband Zechariah, himself a priest, that is the New Testament's sole infertility narrative. It forms a bridge between the Old and New Testament, as well as between biblical times and ours, and is therefore a fitting subject for our final chapter.

We leave the Old Testament on a happy note, and will enter the New Testament and conclude our story on a happy note. This is fitting for reflections inspired by the Bible and life, which from the perspective of faith, begin and end on a happy note.

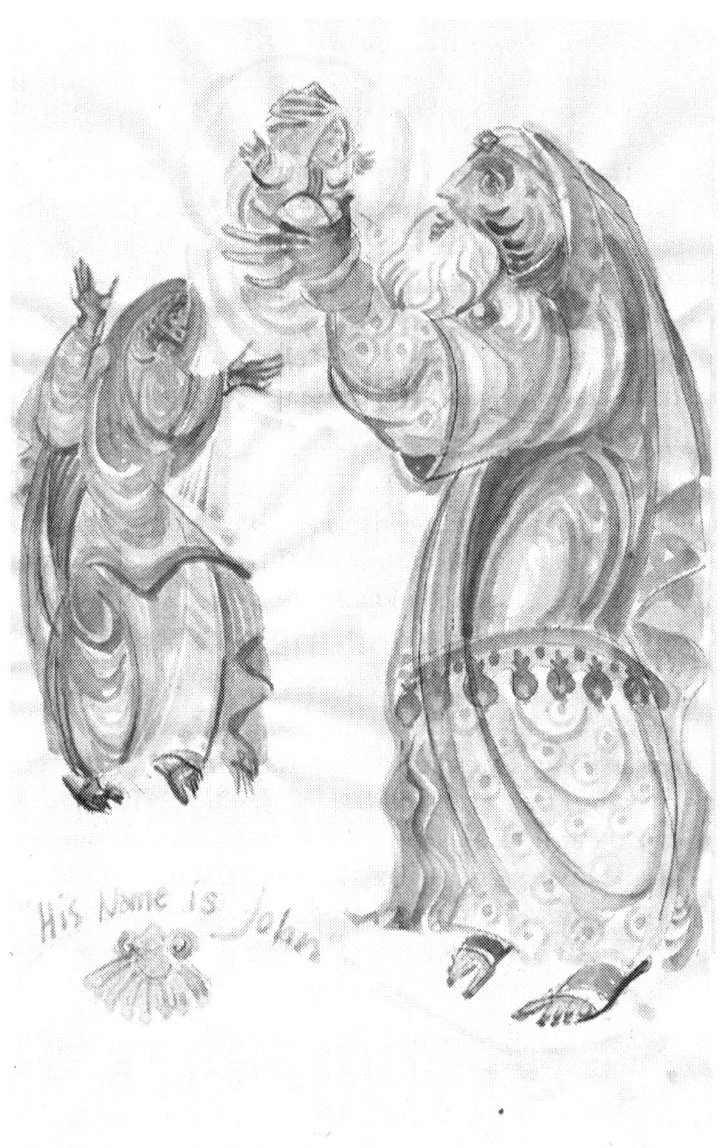

Figure 8. Elizabeth and Zechariah.

It is fitting to end our illustrations with Elizabeth and Zechariah, relatives of those with whom we began, Mary and Joseph. Parallels to their situation are illustrated deftly by the evangelist Luke, who contrasts the honoring of Mary with the mysterious punishment of Zechariah.

On the surface, the mystified response of both seems equally understandable. Mary has not engaged in marital relations, and Elizabeth is past child-bearing age. With regards to Zechariah and Elizabeth, the plight of Sarah and Abraham come to mind, one difference being that Abraham is silenced by Sarah (he goes to God for a solution to her rivalry with Hagar) while Zechariah is muted by the angel. In both cases, God implements His plan for the welfare of all.

Zechariah takes his lumps like a man, and does as he is told, like Mary's husband, Joseph. Zechariah is willing to obey the command of the angel despite his punishment and the well-meaning prodding of friends and relatives. Joseph takes Mary as his wife even though the painful thoughts of her apparent adultery are fresh in his mind. He takes the child and his mother to and from Egypt while remaining in harm's way.

Both men exhibit courage in stepping out in faith according to the Lord's word. They are faithful in deed, while their wives are faithful in words and disposition. God does not provide a road map for any of them, just signs along the way. Divine guidance typically comes to us in a piecemeal, progressive manner that requires us to trust and be patient. In the language of the psalms, it is waiting upon and walking with (in the New Testament, following) the Lord.

Elizabeth humbly and joyfully greets and honors Mary just as the angel did, even though Mary is the younger cousin, and thus according to that culture should be deferential. Elizabeth accepts Zechariah's silent communication that the child's name is to be John. Likewise the Bible records no words between Joseph and Mary. These holy and wise couples remind us that there are ways to communicate beyond words. Joseph and Zechariah are men of few words and loud actions.

It is interesting and instructive that these men are silent partners in their marriages. Scripture focuses primarily on the relationship between their wives. We know that in a matriarchal culture such as the United States far greater attention is paid to the mother than the father. Phone lines overload on Mother's day, while on Father's day usage does not approach capacity.

Scripture challenges us with these questions, among others:

Are husbands willing to humble themselves, give appropriate honor and gratuitous love to their wives, acting mercifully and compassionately towards them while accepting courageously and with integrity the challenges placed before them?

Are wives willing to respect and submit to their husband's judgment, prioritizing them over outside influences while accepting their spiritual guidance and reflecting lovingly upon both the positive and negative examples they set?

When a husband and wife stay united amid the trials and vicissitudes of life, their love can be fruitful in ways beyond their imagining, known only to the mind and providence of God.

Chapter Seven

God's Time is the Right Time

Elizabeth and Zechariah were an elderly infertile Jewish couple living in the Holy Land in the beginning of the first century. Zechariah was a priest and Elizabeth was a descendant of Aaron, the first Jewish priest.

In a scene familiar to us from the Old Testament, an angel appears to Zechariah and announces that his wife will bear a son whom Zechariah is to name John. Zechariah responds the same way Abraham and Sarah did, and in a similar manner to Mary, the mother of Jesus, when she received a prophecy of her miraculous pregnancy. However, the angel construes Zechariah's need for confirmation as a lack of faith, and consequently announces that he is going to be struck dumb temporarily.

The angel mentions that his words will be fulfilled in their time, that is, God's time, which is the theme I have chosen for this final chapter. God's time brings suffering, healing, and joy, as we will see in the story of Zechariah and Elizabeth. God's time is intimately tied to the mystery of both procreation and potential fulfillment, as it is at the root of our capacity to give and develop life. We can bear the unbearable more peacefully when we remember and trust that God's time is the right time for relieving us of our burden, and that Jesus makes our burden lighter paradoxically by inviting us to share in his (cf. Mt 11:28-30).

Why the Dumb Stunt?

On first glance, the punishment received by Zechariah seems a bit arbitrary and harsh. From our perspective, his response to the angel's announcement was natural, and certainly not disrespectful. Who among us wouldn't be perplexed, fearful, and skeptical? Neither religion nor experience prepares us for this kind of announcement.

Further, the Bible reports that both Zechariah and Elizabeth were righteous, law-observing Jews. The angel came to bring good news and leaves with Zechariah bereft of his speech. What gives, God? How would you expect him to respond, especially since his initial response to the angel's appearance was terror?

A universal biblical truth that we can apply to this passage is that God doesn't need to explain Himself to human beings. Jesus never tried to justify God's ways to humans. St. Paul references the prophet Isaiah in asserting that the clay has no right to demand an accounting from the potter (cf. Rom 9:20-22; Isa 45:9-11). Job learned the folly of trying to do so (cf. Job 38:1-3; 40:1-5). God is happy to indulge our questions, frustrations, and anger, but He does not have to answer to us nor make His ways understood.

God's sovereignty is very difficult for people in a democratic and science-oriented society to stomach. We want to know why events transpire as they do, and we think persons in authority are accountable to provide answers.

On a personal level, it is difficult to reconcile a loving God with our inability to bear children or develop ourselves and the world. Why would God give a command and then stand idly by while it is made inaccessible by nature or the sinful or foolish actions of ourselves or others born more out of weakness and ignorance than malice? For the same reason He is harsh with someone who is incredulous when told that a dream that he has been denied all these years will miraculously come true. Only God knows.

The biblical rationale for suffering, human abuse of free will, is comprehensible intellectually and morally but not emotionally or experientially. The only fully satisfactory answer to suffering is a person, not a concept. The Gospels emphasize Jesus' complete freedom in accepting not only his own innocent suffering, but the suffering of all persons throughout history.

Jesus never tried to justify or explain suffering. He debunked some of the popular theories (cf. Jn 9:1-3; Lk 13:1-5), but his main teaching was by example, thereby setting a precedent for us. He taught about suffering through proverbs, parables, and personal encounters, but in an open-ended, personal way that engaged rather than coerced his audience:

> "Behold my servant, whom I uphold, my chosen, in whom my soul delights; I have put my Spirit upon him, he will bring forth justice to the nations. He will not cry or lift up his voice, or make it heard in the street; a bruised reed he will not break, and a dimly burning wick he will not quench; he will faithfully bring forth justice. He will not fail or be discouraged till he has established justice in the earth; and the coastlands wait for his law" (Isa 42:1-4).

In an address to disabled persons in 1964, Pope Paul VI commented that the capacity for love is equivalent to the capacity for suffering. We are willing to endure much for those we care for. Our deeds, more than our words, reveal what is in our heart.

There comes a point when we need to balance our wrestling with God with a willingness to accept His will and timing, even when it contradicts ours. This is a life-long struggle, and we should be patient with ourselves as we learn how to live with God and His mysterious ways.

Am I willing to move on with my life amid uncertainty, disappointment, and disillusionment and allow God His sovereignty, that is, the right to order life as He wills without having to answer to me? How difficult it is to subordinate our ego, fears, and agenda, and trust that God will act with our best interests in mind. Easy to preach, tough to practice.

When I surrender to God in this way, what typically occurs? What experiences come to mind?

When I deny God His sovereignty by rebelling against His will or my situation, what typically results? What experiences come to mind?

God Expects A Lot of His Gifted Children

Inexplicable actions on the part of God or His angelic messengers in the Bible often have symbolic meanings that are lost or only partially comprehensible to future generations. Another possible explanation for Zechariah's punishment is that while his culpability escapes us, God sees room for improvement, and thus issues a corrective. As a priest, Zechariah would have been familiar with the story of Sarah and Abraham and the other infertile couples in the Old Testament, and thus perhaps should have seen a precedent and been more receptive. Of course, this is said in hindsight and without knowing what it feels like to encounter an angel and receive a fantastic prophesy.

The Bible and the people of its era are much more comfortable with both divine and human discipline than we are (cf. Heb 12:5-13). We moderns have done a marvelous job of inverting the religious relationship and fashioning God in our image, which in the Bible is referred to as idolatry.

God does not coddle us, particularly those to whom He has given much:

> "From everyone to whom much has been given, much will be required; and from the one to whom much has been entrusted, even more will be demanded" (Lk 12:48).

Psalm 8 is a marvelous testimony to the potential and responsibilities God has entrusted to us:

> "When I look at your heavens, the work of your fingers, the moon and the stars that you have established; what are human beings that you are mindful of them, mortals that you care for them? Yet you have made them a little lower than God, and crowned them with glory and honor. You have given them dominion over the works of your hands; you have put all things under their feet, all sheep and oxen, and also the beasts of the field, the birds of the air, and the fish of the sea, whatever passes along the paths of the seas" (Ps 8:3-8).

Each person is a gifted child of God. One of the purposes of prayer, dialogue, and cooperation with others, particularly believers, is for each of us to discover and develop our gifts. Obstacles to our potential fulfillment, such as we have discussed throughout this book, should not influence us to give up and let our gifts lie dormant. Such obstacles are often a good sign, as they indicate that we are meeting resistance from the forces of mediocrity and negativity within us and society.

Each of us has to discern through prayer, study, counsel, and experience how we are to use our gifts, and whether obstacles and setbacks indicate a need for a change in tactics or direction. Often it is best to stay the course, to do what we are doing, to persevere. If we had a good reason for embarking on a path, we ought to let things develop until we receive convincing evidence of a need for an alternate approach.

If it was easy to develop our gifts, we'd either be extraordinarily blessed, the recipient of good timing and circumstances, or we'd be conforming to the mediocre and often destructive ways of the world. Many persons who contributed much to their own and subsequent generations met resistance in their day and only received their due posthumously.

For example, St. Thomas Aquinas was not held in the same esteem in his day that he has been by subsequent generations. St. John of the Cross, one of Christianity's finest teachers of mystical prayer, was jailed by his religious order. St. Joan of Arc was burned at the stake by the very people she helped liberate. Jesus was rejected by the people He came to save and was crucified for his perceived unorthodoxy. The prophets before him likewise met rejection and persecution (cf. Lk 6:22-23).

While we may not achieve notoriety in subsequent generations, it is God's opinion that counts most. By striving to fulfill our procreative and development potential, even amid seemingly insurmountable obstacles, we act as faithful stewards of the gifts He has given us. Mother Teresa of Calcutta's words continually come to mind: God does not ask us to be successful, but faithful. Our ultimate accountability will be to God:

> "Think of us in this way, as servants of Christ and stewards of God's mysteries. Moreover, it is required of stewards that they be found trustworthy. But with me it is a very small thing that I should be judged by you or by any human court. I do not even judge myself. I am not aware of anything against myself, but I am not thereby acquitted. It is the Lord who judges me. Therefore do not pronounce judgment before the time, before the Lord comes, who will bring to light the things now hidden in darkness and will disclose the purposes of the heart. Then each one will receive commendation from God" (1 Cor 4:1-5).

St. Paul's affirmation of our active role in the salvation of the world reminds us that both individually and collectively God thinks and expects a lot of us:

> "I am now rejoicing in my sufferings for your sake, and in my flesh I am completing what is lacking in Christ's afflictions for the sake of his body, that is, the church" (Col 1:24).

According to Christian thought, Jesus' afflictions and death resulted in the reconciliation of the world to God (cf. 2 Cor 5:18-21). Our "completing what is lacking" refers to our uniting our sufferings with his, thereby fulfilling our part of his mission and making us participants in his saving actions.

Do I believe that God thinks and expects a lot of me and my loved ones? What experiences have influenced my perception of this? How would I like my perception to grow?

Do I believe that I contribute to the world's salvation when I refuse to give up or become embittered by my sufferings, and instead love God, neighbor, and myself as best I can?

What are my gifts?

What are the main obstacles to the utilization and sharing of my gifts?

What do I discern is the right way for me to respond to these obstacles? Should I persevere in my course, make minor or significant alterations, or try another path?

Sometimes a way is completely closed to us, and for practical purposes we have little choice but to choose another path. However, this path may not be blocked in the future, and we can always use our gifts at a later time.

Do I support others in using their gifts?

Do I recognize that children are a gift from God, like other potentialities, and that if I am not gifted with them in the present, I should not close myself to other paths of life-giving? As discussed in chapters one and two, these include adoption, outreach to the elderly or disadvantaged children, other community service activities, and development of my own and others' potential.

Do I take quiet time daily to discern God's initiative in my life and His guidance as to how to use my gifts properly?

Do I truly believe that through faithfulness in small matters entrusted to me (cf. Mt 25:14-30; Lk 16:10) I can play an important role in the salvation of the world? What experiences and beliefs influence my attitude and actions in this regard?

Time in Seclusion

After conceiving, Elizabeth goes into seclusion. There was no legal or religious reason for this, so it seems fair to attribute a social or spiritual purpose to it. The Bible's silence invites us to use our experience, intuition, and reasoning to determine the relevance of this behavior for us.

I think that Elizabeth was a bundle of emotions. She needed time to adjust, as she and Zechariah were no spring chickens. Perhaps she needed time to sort through her emotions with God, who had withheld the gift of infertility for so long and had finally delivered.

Elizabeth also probably worried about what other people would think, given her advanced age. After all, it had been a millennium (Hannah and Elkanah) since such miraculous pregnancies had occurred in Israel. However, the joy of an expectant mother would transcend any sensitivity to community opinion.

When I experience the intense pressures of biological or functional infertility, or find myself delivered from it, I may find myself needing time apart. Social pressures and influences can be stifling and overwhelming, and I may need time alone or with my partner and family.

Perhaps I feel the need to reconnect with God. I may have drifted from Him and become embittered by all the heartaches and disappointments. I need exclusive reconciliatory time with God. I can't get close to Him and hear His message when I am continually distracted by external noises and chaotic activity.

Do I need quiet, perhaps even secluded, time? What steps can I take to attain it?

What benefits have I received when I took time apart in the past, whether on a small or significant scale?

Do loved ones in my midst need secluded time? How might I facilitate this for them? Do we need it together, perhaps a vacation to relax, recharge our batteries, and rediscover each other anew?

Identifying with People in Pain

Identifying with biblical characters can refine our empathy and help us be more sensitive to persons who are grieving and rejoicing in our midst, including ourselves. However, when ascribing motives to biblical characters, we inevitably project our own experience, beliefs, and bias, and thus we should not impose our applications on others. We can share our perspective without conveying it as dogma.

Elizabeth and Zechariah have been impeded from fulfilling their procreative potential. They likely experienced social rejection as well, given that society's negative outlook on infertility. The fact that Zechariah was a priest, a leader of the people, would have made their infertility all the more conspicuous.

Elizabeth utters words of gratitude and relief that call to mind Sarah's (cf. Gen 21:6-7) and Rachel's (cf. Gen 30:23):

> "This is what the Lord has done for me when he looked favorably on me and took away the disgrace I have endured among my people" (Lk 1:25).

This sheds light on her mind set during her seclusion.

Elizabeth was filled with thanksgiving and relief. God has acted. She manifests the proper response for a believer in the wake of good news: she praises God for His gracious gifts. Of course she had the angel's announcement to go on, and people of that culture attributed significant events ultimately to God, but she still could have injected her own ego into the equation, lamenting that it took too long and that she and her husband deserved better.

When rays of light shine through our agony, we should recall the source of our joy:

> "Every generous act of giving, with every perfect gift, is from above, coming down from the Father of lights, with whom there is no variation or shadow due to change" (Jas 1:17).

What gifts, events, or developments might I give thanks for?

What words would I like to share with God or individuals who cooperated with God in easing my suffering?

What persons in my midst would benefit from my presence and support amid their pain or joy?

With what persons would I like to share my joy or grief on a deeper level? Am I willing to risk rejection by telling them of my need and desire?

Social Stigmas

The second half of Elizabeth's response: "This is what the Lord has done for me when he looked favorably on me and took away the disgrace I have endured among my people" (Lk 1:25) reminds us of the social stigma associated with infertility and how this was felt intensely by the woman. What a burden Elizabeth and to a lesser extent Zechariah must have felt all those years. How many Elizabeths there are in our midst, people laboring under intense physical, psychological, economical, social, and spiritual burdens.

For example, children with a chronic, perhaps life-shortening affliction, and their parents. Adult children taking care of elderly parents and having to make the dreaded nursing home decision. A spouse holding on to a marriage with an irresponsible partner. An abandoned spouse trying to make it alone in a social and economic setting far different than they are accustomed to.

There are equally compelling social stigmas in our day. For example, unemployment, substandard housing, a criminal record, divorce, receiving government subsidies, and being accused of a sexual or family-related crime—with all the sensationalism surrounding these issues, the public generally associates accusation with guilt, and reputations undergo irreparable damage, often without justification.

While Elizabeth's burden and stigma was due to infertility, which because of scientific and social advances is no longer looked upon as a cause for shame, we can substitute our affliction(s) for hers and enter into her experience as a springboard to communicating our pain, hopes, and gratitude to God and others.

At various times we may not be able to relate to Elizabeth's joy. Although we rejoice for her and for ourselves and others when we have reason to celebrate, we also are sad for the part of ourselves and others that remains unfulfilled, for the prayers that go unanswered and the efforts that don't bear fruit. In chapter four we saw how common an experience this is in the Bible and life.

What burdens have I labored under for longer than I like to remember? How have I grown, healed, or regressed through these experiences?

In what experiences have I felt the painful repercussions of social stigmas? Have I asked for God's help in coping and healing, and if so, what has been His response?

How might I ease others' (particularly loved ones') burdens and help them cope with social stigmas? Am I willing to go against cultural values and conventions and stand up for what and who I believe in?

How might I contribute to the mitigation of a social stigma through political or community action?

In what ways do I contribute to the negative effects of social stigmas by going along with the crowd and acting in a prejudiced, judgmental manner?

God's Timing

Most of us are familiar with the story of the Annunciation, that is, the angel Gabriel's announcement to Mary of her divinely infused pregnancy. Mary learns that she is about to bear a special child who will deliver Israel. Mary wonders how this will come about because she has not yet had relations with Joseph. The angel tells her that God will bring about the pregnancy, and that her cousin Elizabeth is also pregnant. She therefore has someone with whom to share her joy. How good it is that God provides companions for our journey. Hopefully, we will seek them out, and both we and they will be responsive.

The angel tells Mary that Elizabeth is now in her sixth month, so apparently God has coordinated things such that Elizabeth has gotten her seclusion out of her system and is ready to spend time with Mary, who certainly could use someone to share her secret with.

Amid troubling circumstances, it is very difficult to believe that God's time is the right time, and that He coordinates human activities in a beneficial way. That is the underlying affirmation of Gabriel's visit to Mary. Using historical and theological analysis, we could speculate as to why God chose that particular time to intervene decisively in human history, but only God knows His real reasons

Likewise, we can try to understand why events have developed in our lives as they have, and what meaning we can ascribe to them, presuming we recognize God's involvement in them. However, we will always be operating on faith rather than sight (i.e., sensate experience; cf. 2 Cor 5:7).

Why Me, Lord?

I have never had much success understanding why God has chosen to permit obstacles to my fulfillment. During soothing and insightful moments of prayer, I may get an inkling, but then I am awakened to the bitter aspects of reality, and doubt creeps in.

I can postulate reasons as to God's timing in certain events, why He comes to my aid one moment and seems to abandon me the next, but that doesn't change the reality. So, I have learned to make the best of things, and hopefully be more insightful, prudent, patient, and compassionate in the process.

In many respects, I don't like my reality. I can identify with the many parts of the Old Testament (e.g., Psalms, Job, Jeremiah) which speak of God's seeming inactivity amid the prosperity of the wicked: Jer 20:7-18, Job 24:12, and Psalms 31, 37, 44, 69, 73, and 77 are among my favorites.

In terms of modern applications, I see many needy people denied government aid while wealthy professional sports franchises are subsidized despite public disapproval. The rich get richer and the poor get crushed amid society's ambivalence.

However, because of my belief in God's initiative I trust that God will work things out in His time, with the suffering of the innocent being coped with humanely by each person's decision to love and act justly and mercifully (cf. Mic 6:6-8), as St. Joseph did when he was confronted with Mary's apparent adultery (cf. Mt 1:18-19). By moving from judging myself and others to mercy, I find peace (cf. Jas 2:13).

Further, I occasionally have glimpses of God's splendid timing, moments when I perceive that He comes through in marvelous fashion. These experiences keep me going, and I return to them during down times for encouragement and consolation.

What is your experience of God's timing? Have you discussed your perspective with God? What kind of message do you receive when you bring it to His attention?

How have you benefited from God's timing? With hindsight can you observe how delays, denials, or initially undesired outcomes might have been in your best interest?

Hope in God

"For nothing will be impossible with God" (Lk 1:37).

When I am deeply discouraged and at the end of my patience, I remember the angel's testimony to God's power. Two persons intimately familiar with excruciating suffering, Job (cf. Job 42:2) and Jesus (cf. Mt 19:26), likewise affirmed God's unlimited capacity to accomplish His plan.

Frankly, I have undergone too many enduring disappointments to expect the miraculous. I'm not about to get my hopes up when I have abundant experiences of not having them fulfilled. This may not be the kind of rhetoric found in most inspirational books, but it's reality for most people. However, even if I do not experience the miraculous, there is still cause for hope.

There are times when God comes through in spectacular fashion. There are plenty of examples of couples getting pregnant when medically such does not seem possible. Patients endure or recover from diseases diagnosed as terminal or injuries deemed debilitating. People overcome huge odds to fulfill some aspect of their potential. For example, an athlete comes back from a serious disease or injury and surpasses all expectations, including his previous standards.

At first I don't think such inspiring stories have anything to do with me. I certainly don't have a tale like that... Or do I?

Considered from societal standards, my life story is rather bland. Like anyone, I could share emotional aspects that might evoke a few tears, but overall my journey has been rather unspectacular. However, on closer inspection, I do have much to draw encouragement and consolation from, as do each of us.

I have overcome major obstacles and setbacks, persevered in discouraging circumstances, put myself in a position to make breakthroughs in various areas, made improvements in many aspects of my life, developed relationships in a healthy manner, and held onto my beliefs and values despite considerable resistance from internal and external forces.

So although it's not enough to make a movie about, it gives me reason for hope. Not only God but plenty of human beings helped me along the way, beginning with loved ones. I am sure you could look at your life and arrive at similar conclusions about your achievements and development.

Consider writing down your recollections and reflections in order to reawaken your awareness, gratitude, and motivation.There have been good and bad times, but I have been fortunate enough to have my primary needs met. God provides enough for me to get by and do what I need to do. St. Paul observed that if we have food and clothing we have all we need (cf. 1 Tim 6:8). As a tent-maker on the go, he wouldn't think of the other necessity, lodging, in the same way as we would.

Trusting in God and accepting what you have rather than what you want, particularly when according to contemporary standards of justice you deserve more, is not an easy way to live. It is certainly not our preference, but it stretches us and keeps us from pride and complacency. We end up accomplishing more than we thought possible.

I view this day-to-day survival mode as God's way of giving me the daily sustenance I pray for in the Lord's Prayer. It keeps my trust centered on God rather than on myself or others. We know how fallible and vulnerable we are, even with the best of intentions.

Thank God and Others

Having the basic necessities of life is already reason for gratitude, but I can also engage in activities and enjoy comforts that three-fourths of the world could only dream of. So, before I start feeling too bad about all I do not have and the many wrongs I have endured (while committing plenty myself), I ought to pay attention to the many blessings that I have, many of which I have received rather than earned.

I have my health, family, friends, freedom, and opportunities to grow personally and professionally. I don't live in fear of forces beyond my control, and I can practice my religion without any interference. Many people cannot say that.

God's Subtle Ways

Along with these blessings, I have been frustrated in many procreative and potential fulfillment efforts. I have learned not to expect the spectacular from God, because when such does occur it usually comes as a surprise. However, I have continually experienced His initiative in small, subtle, but nonetheless significant ways. With the aid of prayer and reflection, I can discover the same divine presence in my present situation, no matter how much reason for discouragement there is.

When God visited the despairing Elijah on Mt. Sinai, He was not in the earthquake, fire, or wind storm, natural signs that the ancients associated with God. He was in the still, small voice (cf. 1 Kings 19:12).

When we are struggling with biological and functional infertility, it is more likely that we will experience subtle rather than grandiose signs from God. One advantage of the subtle sign is that it doesn't overwhelm or distract us from doing everything we can to address our difficulties. We are less likely to get a big head and become presumptuous or complacent and expect the sensational on an ongoing basis.

Using Job as a model (cf. Job 27:5-6), I can persevere in my integrity while maintaining a reasonable degree of cheerfulness. By being attentive to my duties, I put myself in a position to cooperate with God's wondrous interventions that would otherwise escape my notice. If I believe, like Mary, that nothing is impossible with God, I may not achieve my goals in the area of biological and functional fertility, but I'll never stop trying.

I have shared some of my potential fulfillment story and how God and others have helped me along the way. Consider writing your own recollections and reflections on your journey, and its bearing on your procreative and potential fulfillment efforts today.

What experiences and beliefs have influenced your attitude about God's capacity and desire to act in subtle but significant ways in your life?

Do you solicit and reciprocate the support of others, so that you cooperate fully with God in making the marvelous happen?

Sharing Our Story

Shortly after receiving news of her pending pregnancy from the angel, Mary set out in haste to visit Elizabeth. She couldn't wait to share her news and her joy over Elizabeth's unexpected development. She wouldn't let a journey keep her from sharing the moments.

When we embark on a new path in life, or find an obstacle removed from our way, we naturally want to share our joy with loved ones. We likewise feel ecstatic when a loved one finds a door opening to them or a longtime dream being fulfilled. We fill up with such emotion that we sense that if we don't share it we are liable to burst.

Not everyone has loved ones to share their news with. There are times when we don't have someone to commiserate or celebrate with. There are also times when due to shame, shyness, or stubbornness we don't avail ourselves of the opportunity to share with others. Mary's enthusiastic rendezvous with Elizabeth reminds us of the importance of dealing with our fertility and potential fulfillment adventure in a communal rather than isolated manner. In few circumstances do we need each other as much as when our ability to procreate or utilize our gifts is impeded or fulfilled.

Do I share my joys and pains with appropriate persons, and welcome their news and feedback? If I am reluctant, why? How might I overcome any excessive inhibitions?

Do I make myself available and communicate receptivity to those who would share their story with me? What underlies any refusal to be accessible?

No Competition

Elizabeth and Mary present a refreshing contrast to Sarah and Hagar and Rachel and Leah. They form a community rather than a competition. They defer to each other rather than try to go one up. They remind us of the limitations of gender generalizations and cultural perceptions. Not all women respond to feminine counterparts in potentially competitive situations in a catty, adversarial fashion. Likewise some men freely ask directions, admit they're wrong, or go to counseling when they have a problem.

Elizabeth and Mary are secure persons who are as interested in others as in themselves. They feel spontaneous joy for others. How liberating it is to desire the good of others and not be preoccupied with our own situation. This is particularly therapeutic amid experiences of loss and deprivation, when our tendency is to close in upon ourselves. Elizabeth and Mary remind us that it is possible to approach our problems in a communal, cooperative manner, and to be humble and gracious rather than haughty and resentful.

Am I overly or inappropriately competitive in any areas or with any persons? What drives me to be like this? How might I modify this tendency?

In what areas or with whom am I cooperative and collegial? How might I bring this attitude and behavior to other areas and relationships?

God Works in Mysterious Ways

When I was young, my mother always told me that God works in mysterious ways, and I continually experience that. The stories we have reflected on, both in the Bible and in our lives, are prime examples.

Suffering is the scene of God's most mysterious actions. Mother Teresa was around suffering more than most people, and one of her most frequent exhortations was that we should not automatically view suffering as punishment. Rather, it is God's call to love as He does, freely and unconditionally.

When we take up this challenge, even though we fall short, we cannot help but journey towards our procreative and functional potential fulfillment. The more we emulate God, the more life-giving we become and the closer we come to our true selves, the person God made us to be.

What father is unmoved by pleas for mercy from his children? Instead of trying to justify ourselves and determine to what degree we and others are right or wrong in particular situations, we can leave that to God and simply ask His forgiveness and help. God wants to bless us, but His ways of doing so are usually not according to our agenda. That's what makes life a spiritual adventure even when the material dimension of our lives is frustrating and impoverished.

The Bible reports that when Elizabeth had her son, her neighbors and relatives viewed it as a sign of God's mercy and rejoiced with her. Instead of viewing our losses and deprivations as punishments and indications of God's displeasure, we should look on them as opportunities to grow in virtues such as patience, faith, love, wisdom, courage, compassion, and perseverance, and to allow God to make our experience revelatory and redemptive for others as well, as in the case of Zechariah.

Consider the puzzling episode of Zechariah's dumbness. We, and perhaps he as well, may remain clueless as to precisely what his offense was, and how he was more culpable than other biblical persons confused by an angel's fantastic announcement. However, the way the story turns out, we discover that Zechariah's offense was used by God to bring about His wonderful plan:

> "We know that all things work together for good for those who love God, who are called according to his purpose" (Rom 8:28).

Zechariah's dumbness became a vehicle not only for his expression of obedience—in accordance with the angel's directive, he wrote "his name is John"—the loosening of his tongue became a sign for the people that loosened lips throughout the land. True word of mouth advertising! God can correct our flaws and turn them into manifestations of His love and power.

We should also note that the story concludes with Zechariah's hymn of praise, which in style and language resembles Mary's. This is the Bible's way of setting them together as two compliant spirits, in this case the latter more obedient than the former, but both seeking to serve the Lord. Zechariah's hymn reminds us that we can overcome difficulties and detours on our path if we trust in God and do what we think is right, what we believe He asks of us.

Have I experienced a minor mistake or weakness bearing fruit in a disproportionately positive fashion? Could God be behind the transformation of my shortcomings and errors into opportunities for growth? If so, what implications might this have for daily life and my future development?

How might I be gentler and more compassionate and encouraging with myself and others so that mistakes and weaknesses can be more frequently and fluidly turned into occasions of growth and healing for myself and others?

If applicable, why am I unforgiving of imperfections in myself or others? What are the roots of such an attitude?

The Cooperative Couple

Excluding those on a vendetta, people who are cooperative with members of their own sex are usually cooperative with the opposite sex. Elizabeth manifests reciprocality and a communal spirit with her husband, just as she had with Mary.

A cooperative spirit does not mean that you pander to others. Elizabeth is firm about naming the boy John, despite the urging of her relatives and friends and a natural desire to please her husband and provide him with a namesake. It would have been easy to get caught up in the moment and cater to insistent, well-meaning requests. We can admire the strength of character of this woman who accepted the gift of her son without acting in a possessive way. She accepts Zechariah's communication of the angel's instructions and does not introduce her own agenda.

Likewise, Zechariah does not impose his ego onto what unbeknownst to him was a major event in salvation history. He is gracious for God's gift in the way it was given, and does not inject his natural desire for a namesake.

This mature couple present a united front against peer pressure. They are of one heart and purpose, even though Zechariah is prevented from speaking with Elizabeth. I wonder what it was like for them while he was locked in silence. Accommodating themselves to this situation, they communicated volumes through gestures, touch, and actions.

Many couples cannot get along although they share the gift of speech, while without this capacity Elizabeth and Zechariah find a way to manage. They are a model of pliability, teamwork, and resilience. Their secret is their obedience/receptivity to God and each other, and their commitment to their faith, marriage, and child.

Zechariah's silence may have been a factor in Elizabeth's seclusion. Perhaps they decided to give themselves space in preparation for their unprecedented experience. Couples that cooperate closely also need time by themselves.

Elizabeth and Zechariah exemplify mutuality, unity, and obedience. In our prayer and reflection on this passage, we can imagine going to them with our personal or relationship problems, and listening to their response.

Were I to dialogue with Elizabeth and Zechariah, I would ask them how they avoided bitterness, disillusionment, second-guessing, and blaming each other. I believe they would attribute it to mutual love and respect, prayer, quality time together and apart, and the support of their family members, as evidenced by the community's joy at their son's birth.

Knowing that the proof is in the pudding and that love is not a science, I get more of my insights into marriage from long-married couples than from textbooks. I have often asked these couples about their relationship, and I invariably receive answers particular to their situation. There is no one-size-fits-all formula for marital harmony. They acknowledge their blessings and do not judge those who have been unable to stay together. They keep their advice simple, recognizing that each couple must develop their own rules, routines, and patterns.

Elizabeth can identify with the social stigmas and sense of self-doubt that we experience. Zechariah can relate to being singled out for punishment in an obvious, humiliating, and seemingly unjust way. They understand the difficulties of persevering and "hoping against hope" (cf. Rom 4:18), that is, holding onto their dreams and trusting in God's capacity for reversing negative situations and accomplishing His will despite human opposition and unfavorable natural circumstances.

I experience this capacity of God as I discover that the better I write and the more insightfully I speak the more I experience rejection and disappointment. Anyone who pursues the truth will encounter resistance, discouragement, and loneliness.

However, God gives me the strength to keep going. He opens up small doors that enable me to make progress, even if others do not recognize it as such. At 6"7, I hit my head on these doors often, stumbling to accept God's solutions rather than mine. As I pick myself up He puts people in my path to help and encourage me, as well as aggravate and challenge me, and when the time is right, as this chapter's title proclaims, He'll accomplish His purposes, though they may not coincide with mine.

It is not a secure life, but a peaceful, rewarding one. And it is rarely boring. God, like a human lover, knows how to keep us on our toes and spice things up. He blesses us with the capacity to find humor amid our difficulties, and to be cheerful when we feel just the opposite.

How sad it is that not only nuclear family life, but broader family life has broken down in our time. In previous generations couples had a much larger support network for coping with losses and deprivations. Recognizing this, we should band together and support each other with all our might, as more than in any previous era, we may be all we've got.

What would you say to Elizabeth and Zechariah? What questions would you have, and how do you think they would respond?

What parallels can you draw between them and you?

What do Elizabeth and Zechariah have to say to modern couples?

A Modern Elizabeth

My aunt Elizabeth was unable to have children. She and her husband, Frank, were nice folks and cared deeply for each other. They chided me for my interest in the Beatles and other popular groups, urging me to choose Bach not rock.

As I steadfastly rejected such culture, I accepted their gift of an album containing what I referred to as high brow music, and secretly enjoyed it. It contained mellow songs arranged by Jackie Gleason and played by an orchestra under his direction. It would be difficult to get more schmaltzy than that. As a young adult, I played this for my dates to set a romantic mood, only to receive the most incredulous looks. To modify Gleason's trademark expression, "and away they went."

I never asked my aunt and uncle how they coped with their infertility, but I did inquire as to how they were able to get along so well. My uncle Frank was extremely easy-going and affable, which was one obvious explanation for their camaraderie. They had similar interests and compatible personalities. They didn't focus and harp on each other's weaknesses, much less try to change them. Most important, they tried to do for each other, and didn't worry about what others had. Though they didn't have children of their own, they reached out to their nieces and nephews. They prayed for me and always welcomed me into their home.

Who are your Aunt Elizabeth and Uncle Frank, family members or friends who set a good example and help(ed) make life pleasant? Is there anything you can do for them?

What are your dearest memories of them, and how have they influenced you?

John the Baptist and Transitions

A brief reflection on John the Baptist will tie our story together. He was a man of great suffering who bridged two eras. He was a throwback to the Old Testament prophets at the same time that he prepared the way for Jesus. He is relevant to us as we struggle with the many transitions in our life.

The transitions we experience, both personally and collectively, have an effect on our procreative and functional potential fulfillment. Women who are constantly stressed by unending and unpredictable changes in their activities and environment are less liable to conceive than those who live less frenetic lives. A husband who works two or even three jobs may not be around enough to engage in satisfying relations with his wife and children. Persons between jobs face many obstacles not only to exercising their gifts, but making enough to get by. In some relationships, rules change so fast and with little or no notice that we find ourselves giving offense and experiencing repercussions with actions that previously would not only have been considered harmless, but appropriate.

We live in a world that is losing its human values and replacing them with technological ones. Material concerns are superseding the spiritual domain. In popular culture and the business and consumer world, pleasure and privilege (e.g., the unconscionable increase in chief executive salaries since 1980) take precedence over principle. Individual rights, i.e., personal expression and freedom, garner more respect socially than religious observance and moral integrity. Spiritual books are published more for their marketability than their spiritual value. Competition and self-interest has overwhelmed community values and respect for the common good in the consumer society, business world, and political arena. Trust has broken down at every level of society, and security concerns and expenditures are at an all time high.

Such constant and often negative change impedes us from fulfilling our procreative and functional potential by creating an unstable environment not conducive to consistency. We humans are creatures of habit, and when we are continually prevented from settling into steady routines, we have difficulty functioning effectively.

Before we presume that our generation is unique in its moral and developmental chaos, we need to remember John the Baptist's message, environment, and fate. His society had likewise broken down in many ways. Many of the religious leaders had fashioned an uneasy truce with the oppressive government. Society was polarized between the haves and have-nots, between self-proclaimed saints and detested sinners. Roman oppression was omnipresent, and God had been silent lately. He hadn't inspired any biblical books or prophets for over a century. Hearts had grown cold, and the people needed to be woken up, just like us.

John the Baptist was just the person to provide such a wake-up call. He lived an austere life, forsaking staples of Jewish life such as marriage, children, and a comfortable home environment. The common folks listened to him because he lived what he preached.

John never lost sight of his mission or master. He kept his mission from being too closely identified with himself. When Jesus arrived, John gracefully bowed out (cf. Jn 3:25-30), even though he had his doubts (cf. Mt 11:2-6). God requires faith, humility, and trust from His greatest messengers, those who receive His word first hand (cf. Lk 12:48; Jn 14-17; 1 Cor 9:16; Jas 3:1).

John as a Model of Potential Fulfillment

Unfortunately, John crossed one too many influential persons, and exited this world ingloriously. He was imprisoned and then beheaded at the request of an adulterous queen and her stooge daughter. A man of impeccable integrity and morals done in by licentious persons. Isn't that how life often goes? Amazingly, God accomplishes His plan not only in spite of such developments, but through them:

> "Who will separate us from the love of Christ? Will hardship, or distress, or persecution, or famine, or nakedness, or peril, or sword? As it is written, "For your sake we are being killed all day long; we are accounted as sheep to be slaughtered."
>
> No, in all these things we are more than conquerors through him who loved us. For I am convinced that neither death, nor life, nor angels, nor rulers, nor things present, nor things to come, nor powers, nor height, nor depth, nor anything else in all creation, will be able to separate us from the love of God in Christ Jesus our Lord" (Rom 8:35-39).

Jesus gave the ultimate compliment to John the Baptist. He observed that John fulfilled his mission and was true to his identity more than any other person (cf. Mt 11:7-11). Yet, even John's greatness had its limits. Jesus said that the person who followed him with the sincerity of a child was greater than John, meaning that entry into the kingdom of heaven was more important than compliance with the law, though of course the two need not be mutually exclusive.

John is a marvelous inspiration for coping with infertility because he went without children and the comfort of a spouse, and according to Jesus himself served as a model of potential fulfillment.

The moral is, if we trust in God amid our obstacles, we can surpass even John, who did not live to experience the full measure of Jesus' mission. Parents want more for their children than they had, and Jesus promised that his disciples' accomplishments would surpass his because of his intercession (cf. Jn 14:12). Jesus healed by word and touch, but his apostles healed also through their shadow and clothing (cf. Acts 5:15; 19:11-12).

A Dear John Letter

And so, John, you lived a difficult life with few comforts. Because you were born to elderly parents, you probably lost them early in life. As an adult, your time with your cousin Jesus was limited due to your busy schedules and intense missions and adversaries. You probably knew that you both were headed for trouble, as your opposition to societal values and authorities was bound to lead to retaliation and violence. Since you would not fight back, step back, or water down your message, your fate was sealed.

Each of us could compose some variation of this communication to John.

John, I hurt so much from the losses and deprivations I've experienced and observed. I know you understand, because you had your own. I wanted kids and couldn't have them. I tried to adopt and it didn't work out. I've experienced rejection in the most profound way. Family members died before their time. Family members didn't get along at crucial times, and resentments lingered. Some struggled to get by, leading lives far below their potential.

So many doors to my personal and professional growth have been slammed in my face. So many of my dreams have died and opportunities slipped through my fingers. My hope seems limited to getting through the day and awaiting my reward in heaven.

John's Projected Response

Karl, and whoever else may be listening, don't give up or try to be other than you are. No matter how badly you mess up, you can always go home to God. I welcomed many a hardened soldier, tax collector, oversexed person, and jaded religious leader back into God's good graces. I saw many persons whose lives had fallen apart recover through the power of prayer and repentance.

Your path has been painful, and your suffering is far from over. However, you have experienced manifold joy as well. Despite my foreboding message, I never lost sight of life's joys and possibilities. I couldn't stand hypocrisy, and I hope you avoid that route. I lived my message long before preaching it. Never make an idol of popularity or acceptance. I was well known, but it made my life more difficult and deprived me of my beloved solitude and communing with nature.

Tell God what you're feeling, your hopes and dreams that have gone unfulfilled. Thank Him for all He has done for you and your loved ones. Love your loved ones. I had great parents, wonderful aunts and uncles, and a special cousin. I never forgot my roots, and I hope you don't forget yours. Remember to tell your loved ones that you love them, and do what you can to help them cope with their losses and deprivations. Ask God's and others' help in coping with yours. I have faith that you'll make it. I'm praying for you, and I'll put in a good word with my cousin.

Summary: Lessons Gleaned from Elizabeth and Zechariah

The New Testament's bridge to the Old Testament, John the Baptist, was fittingly born to infertile parents. We reflected on the mysterious punishment of Zechariah, John's father, for a response to the angel very similar to that uttered by Mary.

Zechariah is a model for persons who accept perplexing corrections and consequences as part of divine providence with humility and integrity. This does not imply passivity, but responsible obedience and proactivity. Each of us plays a role in God's saving plan, particularly when we persevere amid setbacks and confusion.

As with individuals and couples struggling with and finally overcoming infertility or other obstacles, Elizabeth experienced a range of emotions. We imaginatively accompanied her during Mary's visit (cf. Lk 1:39-45), asking ourselves what they might have discussed, and how they might advise and console us amid our time of waiting.

God's time may be the right time, but we need help in the mean time. Zechariah and Elizabeth can inspire and console us while we wait.

Elizabeth and Zechariah, along with the other biblical couples we have considered in this book, offer compelling examples of hope amid hopelessness and joyful reversals of fortune. They exemplify the importance of living the paradoxical challenge of accepting undesirable situations out of obedience without resigning ourselves passively and irresponsibly to them.

Submission to God's Will

> "Here am I, the servant of the Lord; let it be with me according to your word" (Lk 1:38).

One of the themes of chapter one was obedience, and Mary's classic response helps us come full circle in the book and return to this timeless but counter-cultural topic. It is difficult to emulate Mary in giving God an unconditional yes, to respond affirmatively to His request when you don't know all of its ramifications. You recognize that it will entail uncertainty, rejection, and suffering along with joy, peace, and fulfillment, because that is the nature of life when lived authentically. This is odious to a society that craves security and comfort. In this concluding story, we will consider a modern application of Mary's challenge, and contemplate the various ways we are called to accept it in our individual lives.

Letting Go of Control and Autonomy

Greg and Gloria have tried for years to have a child, and have recently decided to adopt. Because they are Catholic, certain medical procedures such as artificial insemination were morally off limits. Neither understood or agreed completely with the Church's position, but they went along with it and decided to pursue adoption.

Gloria bore considerable resentment towards the Church because she felt that the celibate men who make up the rules on this subject were exceeding their authority and competence. She and Greg discussed it with their parish priest and he was empathetic, but was unable to explain the Church's position in a convincing manner.

Greg and Gloria had several intense arguments on this subject, and Gloria sometimes projected her anger onto other issues, thereby exacerbating minor disagreements or annoyances. However, the bottom line is that Greg and Gloria reconciled on an ongoing basis and followed the Church's teaching, even at great personal cost.

Greg and Gloria practiced obedience on several levels. First, they obeyed each other in the sense of listening respectfully and trying to honor each other's needs. They avoided any kind of distancing, choosing to conflict civilly and make up when problems became too intense.

Second, they obeyed their Church, even when it was not their natural inclination and discerned preference. They achieved inner and interpersonal peace, albeit after much strife, by somehow arriving at an uneasy synthesis of conscience and Church teaching. They accepted the painful and uncertain consequences of their decision and entrusted themselves to the Lord. (Others faced with a similar dilemma might opt for obedience to conscience rather than Church teaching, but the relevant moral issues and subjective considerations exceed this book's scope.)

It can be easy to love God because you don't have to directly face Him or deal with His negative issues. It is quite another challenge to obey a civil or religious authority, parent, teacher, or boss who exercises their authority imprudently, prejudicially, or oppressively.

Greg and Gloria didn't respond as unconditionally as Mary did, but such acts are rare. However, their response was in the spirit of Mary's, which enabled them to identify with Elizabeth and Zechariah and use their example as a starting point for prayer and discernment.

You don't have to identify perfectly with the Bible in order to relate to it. The biblical writers themselves did not employ an exaggerated literalism. They used their source materials in a creative way without distorting the message so that their audience would be able to relate to it.

Through prayer, study, classes, consultation with competent authorities or confidants, and consistent reading, we can learn how to distinguish historical and culturally-conditioned details from the Bible's timeless and personal message.

The Bible can be viewed as a letter from God and other believers designed to facilitate communication with God and others and to evoke a healthy, spiritual response. Each of us encounters the Bible and life in their own way, and we should not feel that a biblical passage has to fit us like a strait jacket, leaving little room for movement. To the contrary, God respects our freedom and sincerity, and wants us to approach Him where we are, rather than where we think we should be.

What does Mary's obedient response have to do with my situation?

In what way can I emulate it?

What are the barriers to my manifesting an obedient response to God and others amid my obstacles, losses, and deprivations?

In the end, there is no absolute remedy for or explanation of biological or functional infertility. All we can do is join Jesus, Mary and Joseph, Job, and the many other biblical heroes and heroines, along with the many good and faithful persons down through the ages as well as in our midst, in persevering in our integrity.

This book is filled with questions because it is in living them, rather than coming up with definitive answers, that we cooperate with God, fellow believers, and persons of goodwill in giving life in the ways available to us. We do so in a manner that embraces this world while looking forward to a better one, where God will wipe away every tear (cf. Isa 25:8; Rev 7:17; 21:4). In this magnificent vocation, you have my prayers and best wishes.

About the Author

Karl A. Schultz is the director of the Genesis Personal Development Center in Pittsburgh, Pennsylvania. He is an author, speaker, and retreat leader on motivational, gender relations, biblical spirituality, time and stress management, wellness, pastoral care, and organizational development topics. He has presented programs in corporate, hospital, hospice, church, association, convention, and retreat environments throughout the United States.

Schultz is one of the world's most prolific authors and teachers of *lectio divina* (holistic spiritual reading), specializing in its applications to suffering, care-giving, lay spirituality, gender relationships (including conflict resolution and coping with infertility), and potential fulfillment topics such as journaling, inner healing, and stress and time management. He has discussed his work on numerous radio and television programs, including the EWTN programs Bookmark, Life on the Rock, and The Abundant Life.

Using the book of Job, Schultz has developed therapeutic and pastoral care applications of *lectio divina* to suffering, care-giving, and infertility, and has presented "Job Therapy" workshops in a variety of health-care, parish, retreat, association, and convention environments. His "Building Up the Human" program was approved by the Pennsylvania Nurses Association for R.N. continuing education accreditation. Schultz has published nine books on applications of biblical spirituality and *lectio divina* to Bible study, suffering, care-giving, stress management, time management, journaling, wellness and potential fulfillment, infertility, and the teachings of Pope Paul VI.

For a listing of other books by the author, reference the bibliography at the front of the book. To purchase books, CDs, or DVDs by Karl A. Schultz, or for information on workshops, retreats, and presentations, contact Genesis Personal Development Center at (412) 766-7545 or at the email address karlaschultz@juno.com. Additional information may be found on the website, karlaschultz.com.

Publisher Information

AMAZON UPGRADE

If you purchased this book from Amazon.com, you can acquire online access via Amazon Upgrade.

ORDERING THIS BOOK IN QUANTITY

Nimble Books does not provide direct fulfillment of individual bookseller or distributor orders. All orders should be placed through our wholesaler, Ingram.

If you are interested in purchasing in quantity (2 or more), we will drop ship for 27.5% discount off list; you pay shipping and handling.

ABOUT NIMBLE BOOKS

Our trusty Merriam-Webster Collegiate Dictionary defines "nimble" as follows:

> 1: quick and light in motion: AGILE *nimble fingers*
>
> 2 a: marked by quick, alert, clever conception, comprehension, or resourcefulness *a nimble mind* b: RESPONSIVE, SENSITIVE *a nimble listener*

And traces the etymology to the 14th Century:

> Middle English nimel, from Old English numol holding much, from niman to take; akin to Old High German neman to take, Greek nemein to distribute, manage, nomos pasture, nomos usage, custom, law

The etymology is reminiscent of the old Biblical adage, "to whom much is given, much is expected" (Luke 12:48). Nimble Books seeks to honor that Christian principle by combining the spirit of *nimbleness* with the Biblical concept of *abundance:* we deliver what you need to know about a subject in a quick, resourceful, and sensitive manner.

Colophon

This book was produced using Microsoft Word and Adobe Acrobat. The cover was produced using The Gimp 2.0.2 with Ghostscript. The cover font is Constantia The spine is Verdana.

Heading fonts and the body text inside the book are in Constantia, chosen because it is a nimble-looking font that is new enough to be fresh on the eyes. Quotations are in Trebuchet MS, a font whose name has nicely medieval connotations.

The American Heritage® Dictionary of the English Language, Fourth Edition, copyright © 2000 by Houghton Mifflin Company defines col·o·phon as follows:

> An ancient Greek city of Asia Minor northwest of Ephesus. It was famous for its cavalry.

Along the same lines, Webster's Revised Unabridged, copyright 1996, 1998, MICRA, Inc.:

> \Col"o*phon\ (k[o^]l"[-o]*f[o^]n), n. [L. colophon finishing stroke, Gr. kolofw`n; cf. L. culmen top, collis hill. Cf. Holm.] An inscription, monogram, or cipher, containing the place and date of publication, printer's name, etc., formerly placed on the last page of a book.

The colophon, then, represents the summit, or fulfillment, of an act of creation, just as Karl's fine book does. I trust and pray that *Bearing the Unbearable* has been a help to you.

Fred Zimmerman

Publisher, Nimble Books LLC

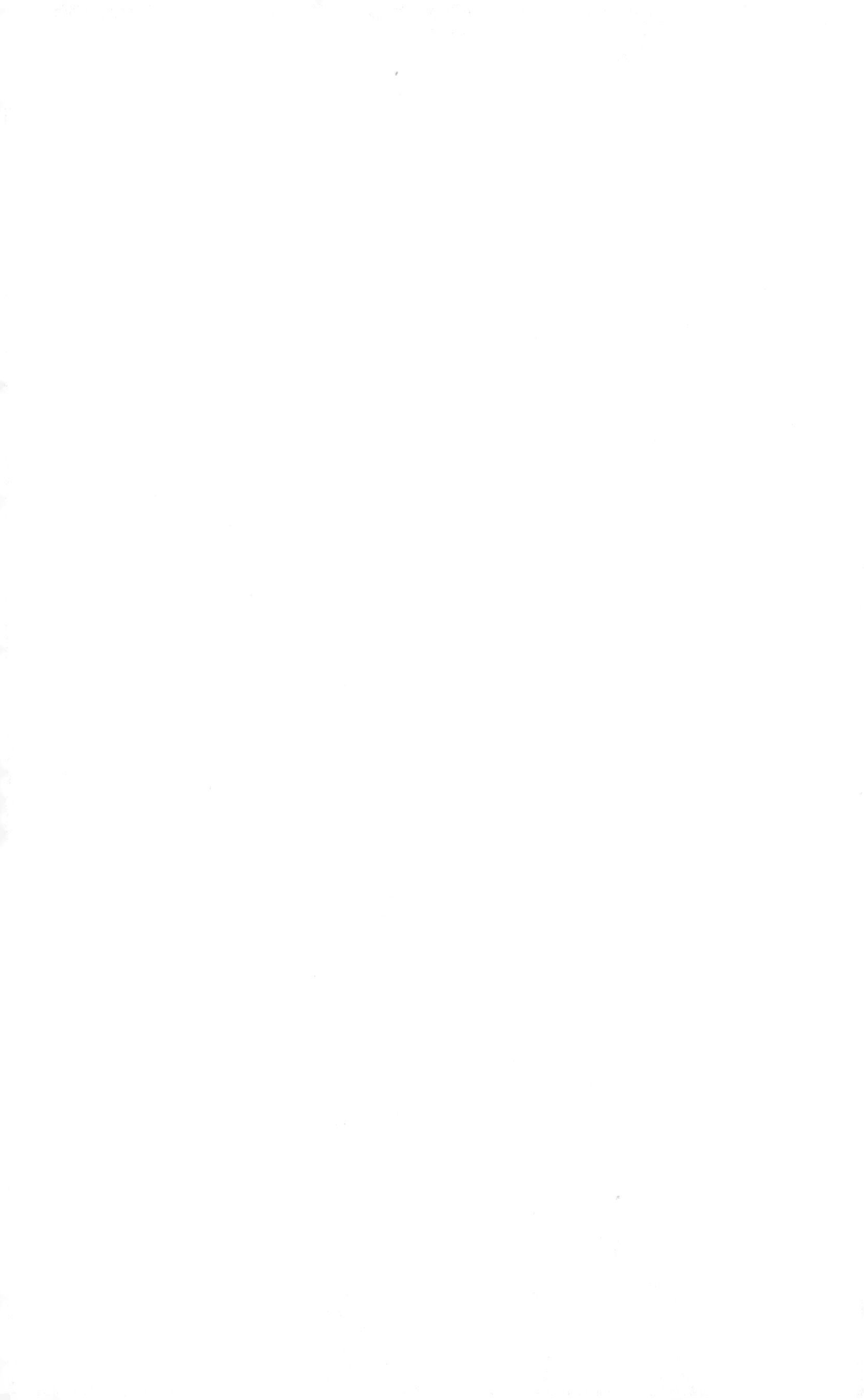

www.ingramcontent.com/pod-product-compliance
Lightning Source LLC
Chambersburg PA
CBHW072307210326
41519CB00057B/3044
9780978813864